Whey Empty Promises

The Surprising Truth about the World's Most Overrated 'Health' Food

By Anthony Colpo

March 2014
Copyright © 2014 Anthony Colpo
All rights reserved worldwide.

Lulu Publishing

ISBN 978-1-304-94083-4

Medical Disclaimer

The contents of this book are presented for information purposes only and are neither intended as medical advice nor to replace the advice of a physician or other health care professional. Anyone wishing to embark on any dietary, drug, exercise or lifestyle change for the purpose of preventing or treating a disease or health condition should first consult with a competent health care professional.

The decision to utilize any information in this book is ultimately at the sole discretion of the reader, who assumes full responsibility for any and all consequences arising from such a decision. The author and publisher shall remain free of any fault, liability, or responsibility for any loss or harm, whether real or perceived, resulting from use of information in this book.

Financial Disclosure

The author does not, and never has, received any form of financial assistance from industry groups that may stand to benefit from the information presented in this book. This includes those from the meat, egg, dairy, nutritional supplement, food, beverage, drug, and agriculture industries. The author does not hold, trade, or speculate in the stock of companies from the aforementioned industries.

Table of Contents

Part I	6
Part II	40
References	77
Free Excerpt from *The Fat Loss Bible*	86
References from Bonus Chapter	107
About the Author	111

Part I

The late Ernest G. Ross once wrote: *"About almost any subject, there are the facts 'everyone knows' and then there are the real ones."*

Ross was referring to those snippets of wisdom that have been repeated so often most people simply assume they're true, but when one starts searching for actual evidence it quickly becomes apparent *there is none*. Here are a few such gems:

Red meat is bad for you. Vegetarians live longer. Saturated fat and high cholesterol levels cause heart disease. Carbs and insulin make you fat.

These are just some of the bromides, incessantly fed to us by the media and so-called 'experts', that I've already dissected in my previous books -- and shown to be totally false.

In this book, I'm going to take another widely-held and cherished mainstream dietary belief, break down its pseudoscientific façade, and expose it for the fallacious nonsense that it is.

Get ready, ladies and gentlemen, as you're about to learn why the belief whole-grain cereals are healthy is a total sham.

History Always Repeats

Before I start dismantling the evidence used by the whole-grain believers to support their pseudoscientific claims, a little history lesson is in order. How, exactly, did this belief that whole-grain cereals are healthier than their refined offspring first come into existence?

That dubious honour falls to one Denis Parsons Burkitt (1911-1993), an Irish-born physician who served as a missionary in Africa during and after World War II. It was there, prior to forming his cereal fibre hypothesis, that Burkitt performed some truly invaluable work and forever stamped his name into medical history. Whilst serving in Uganda in the late 1950s, Burkitt was introduced to a facial tumour that mainly afflicted young children. The severity of the tumours and the lack of effective treatments prompted him to investigate further. During a trip to the UK in 1961, he met Tony Epstein, described his observations, and the two began a collaboration that produced the first electron microscopic evidence of a virus in tumour cells. This eventually led to the discovery of the ubiquitous Epstein-Barr virus, now implicated in a wide variety of disease conditions.

Later in 1961, Burkitt and two colleagues departed on a car journey that would take them more than 10,000 miles around western Africa in a quest to determine the geographic extent of and a possible cause for the virus-induced tumour. Burkitt and his colleagues eventually concluded the virus developed primarily as a result of immune suppression in children with malaria. It was at an international cancer conference in 1963 that the tumour first became commonly known as Burkitt's tumour, a name later modified to Burkitt's lymphoma.

In 1964, Burkitt was able to convince pharmaceutical companies to supply him with chemotherapeutic agents, arguing that his patients offered the chance for a controlled experiment because none had been treated with X-rays. The success of chemotherapy among the African patients was *"amazing,"* with much lower doses required than had been reported for other tumour types[1].

For a lot of African children, Burkitt's compassion and tenaciousness was quite literally a lifesaver.

But then things turned to crap.

Literally.

Epidemiology Throws Us Another Red Herring (Actually, a Brown Herring).

The Burkitt story took a major turn in 1966, when the physician-researcher moved back to England to work with the British Medical Research Council. The following year he met naval Surgeon Captain T. L. Cleave, who believed refined carbohydrate consumption was the cause of many chronic diseases in the West. Cleave shared his theories with Burkitt, and the latter immediately saw parallels with his earlier work on the African lymphoma; namely, that seemingly unrelated diseases may in fact have a common cause.

Aware that certain chronic diseases occurred with much less frequency in Africa than in Western populations, Burkitt applied the same mode of thinking he'd employed when hunting down the cause of the lymphoma. Burkitt's philosophy was that *"one must determine the geographical distribution of a disease...and then seek the environmental factors that are prevalent in areas or groups exhibiting a high frequency of that disease and absent where the disease is rare."* [1]

This process is known as *epidemiology*. The field of epidemiology has been responsible for some truly momentous advancements in public health, such as determining the demographic susceptibility to various infectious diseases and the recognition that smoking was a major cause of lung cancer.

That said, the field of epidemiology has long since degenerated into a data-dredging, cherry-picking free-for-all, one responsible for some of the most absurd and counter-productive nonsense ever contrived in the fields of nutrition and medicine. A classic example is the lipid hypothesis of heart disease, which grew from the early work of Ancel Keys, who cherry-picked small samples of countries then compared their CHD mortality rates in order to create the impression that dietary fat intake and serum cholesterol were related to heart disease. From this fraudulent base, the lipid hypothesis quickly rose to become the cornerstone of modern cardiovascular disease prevention. Its patently false and pseudoscientific nature is readily reflected in the fact that after some five decades of global cholesterol-phobia, CVD still remains the number one killer in the Western world.

As I discussed in *The Great Cholesterol Con*, autopsy studies, decades of randomized clinical trials, and even other epidemiological studies (http://anthonycolpo.com/monica-oh-monica-where-art-thou/) show the lipid hypothesis to be scientifically untenable nonsense. The only 'cholesterol-lowering' treatments that have shown any kind of efficacy are those that also exert other important actions totally independent of cholesterol reduction (for example, statin drugs, partial ileum bypass surgery, and possibly LDL apheresis in FH patients*[1]).

So while epidemiology was undoubtedly of great value in the study of smoking and the demography of infectious diseases, it has repeatedly proved a complete dud for studying relationships between diet and chronic illness. Infectious disease outbreaks tend to be marked by acute and obvious symptoms, and their demographic distribution can hence usually be determined quite quickly. Similarly, the geographic

---

[1] * Statin drugs have been well documented to exert a whole host of pleiotropic actions, including anti-clotting, "anti-inflammatory" and even iron-lowering effects. Partial ileum bypass surgery, employed in the oft-quoted POSCH study, commonly results in weight loss. LDL apheresis in FH patients has been the subject of many favourable case reports, but the RCT evidence is rather shaky; if it is ever proven to work, however, the well-documented reductions in bodily iron stores would be a far more plausible explanation than repeatedly disproved reduction of LDL cholesterol. (http://www.jpands.org/vol10no3/colpo.pdf)

relationship between smoking and lung cancer was so strong, and the likely mechanism so obvious (repeatedly filling your lungs with noxious gases may harm them...duh!), that there was little doubt as to just what researchers were dealing with.

But when it comes to *nutritional* epidemiology, things quickly fall apart. When trying to determine whether a tablespoon of butter each morning will raise a person's risk of heart disease or cancer--conditions that typically take decades to develop and manifest themselves--you'd better be sure the dietary data upon which you are basing your analysis is of very high quality. The dietary data from epidemiological studies, however, is best described as a bad joke. The dietary data in these studies is self-reported, meaning that subjects are given dietary questionnaires, and their answers are assumed to be honest and accurate. Humans being what they are, the reality is that these questionnaires are notoriously prone to misreporting. In fact, as numerous researchers have pointed out, dietary misreporting is not the exception but the *rule* in studies involving self-reported data [2-4].

Sometimes researchers don't even bother with dietary questionnaires, because they've chosen to compare the residents of different countries instead of people living in a certain area of the same country. These types of epidemiological studies are known as *ecological* or *cross-country* comparisons. They rely on nationally reported food intake and disease mortality data, and are the least reliable studies of all because you are comparing apples with oranges: People who not only have different diets but also live under starkly different economic, cultural, political, and environmental conditions.

Ecological comparisons are the very same kind used by Ancel Keys and Denis Burkitt. In fact, the parallels between Keys and Burkitt are quite illustrative. While there is nothing to suggest Burkitt had the duplicitous, ego-driven, bull and bluster personality of Keys (in contrast to the latter, Burkitt really does seem to have been motivated primarily by altruistic motives rather than revenge and self-aggrandizement), both nevertheless relied heavily on dubious epidemiological methods to validate their dietary hypotheses. And both were researchers whose noteworthy prior achievements**[2] allowed their untenable theories to be taken seriously by the reigning health orthodoxy--an orthodoxy that would quite likely have dismissed and even ridiculed lesser known individuals proposing similar theories.

How a Bunch of Crap Inspired the Whole-Grain Theory

The evidence that inspired Burkitt to kick off the fibre phenomenon was a load of crap.

As in, it was literally a load of crap. Burkitt, apparently, had a rather bizarre fascination for human excrement. In addition to the cartoons that graced his

---

[2] **Prior to his shamelessly biased Six and Seven Countries Study, Keys was head researcher of the then ground-breaking Minnesota Study, and a key player in the development of the emergency K-ration in 1942 that was used extensively by U.S. military troops.

articles and book, Burkitt was well known for his collection of photos of human faeces taken on his early morning walks in the African bush. He was reportedly quoted as saying the health of a country's people could be determined by the size of their stools and whether they floated or sank. Seriously. On one occasion he shocked an audience of gastroenterologists by asking, *"How many of you men have any idea of the size of your wives' stools?"*[1]

Yep, this is the same guy who kicked off the worldwide fibre craze, folks.

Burkitt's obsession with doo-doo was fuelled by the observation that increased fibre intake could increase stool weight and reduce stool density, two variables that were *epidemiologically* linked with a reduction in the incidence of several diseases. There was no *clinical* evidence that fibre could reduce the incidence of any disease--and there still isn't--but lack of controlled scientific evidence has never discouraged epidemiologists from pursuing their beloved theories. And Burkitt was certainly no exception in this regard.

Mesmerized by the sterling quality of African faeces, and noting that rural Africans had both a higher fibre intake and a lower incidence of chronic diseases-- including, most notably, colorectal cancer and diverticulitis--Burkitt started putting poo and poo, uh, I mean, two and two together and formed a hypothesis linking fibre intake and chronic disease susceptibility.

Industrialized countries, he noted, had higher rates of chronic disease than developing nations. Therefore, he deduced, some environmental factor that occurs more frequently in industrialized nations must be responsible.

This deduction was perfectly rational, but the line of reasoning Burkitt subsequently embraced was not. To be blunt, it was highly selective and terribly misguided.

Here's why:

Industrialization has been accompanied by a plethora of historically unprecedented physical and psychosocial consequences. People living in highly mechanized societies tend to have regular and unfettered access to an abundance of calorie-dense foods. Meanwhile, their activity levels tend to be far lower than those of their agrarian predecessors, a combination that predisposes to high levels of obesity, which in itself increases the prevalence of various health conditions.

In addition to greater consumption of refined carbohydrates, these populations also begin consuming large amounts of highly processed packaged foods and refined cereal/nut/seed oils, the latter giving rise to unprecedented dietary levels of the omega-6 fatty acid, linoleic acid. Beneficial in small amounts, an overwhelming body of evidence has linked excess amounts of linoleic acid to increased cancer and heart disease incidence.

Sedentary populations tend to spend less time in the sun, and hence their vitamin D levels are lower. Research on vitamin D has exploded over the last dozen or so years, and this research is linking deficiency of this critical vitamin/hormone to an ever-increasing list of health disorders.

Industrialized populations also possess something known as *electricity*, which powers an innovation known as *lighting*, which allows humans to brightly illuminate their surroundings when they would otherwise be dark. This has given humans the ability to greatly suppress natural melatonin release at the flick of a switch and disrupt their all-important circadian rhythms like never before in history. If you're wondering what the heck a *"circadian rhythm"* is, it's the critical 24-hour pattern of hormone release governed by the light-dark cycle that has evolved over millions of years of human evolution.

Your major daily spurt of growth hormone, for example, occurs around 60-90 minutes after falling asleep. However, if you fall asleep in front of the TV with light and noise bombarding your pineal gland, then wake up an hour later and drowsily plod off to bed, you've pretty much sabotaged this key spike in GH. If you keep the house lights shining brightly right up until bedtime, stay up until all hours of the morning surfing the net or watching trashy reality shows, then the light emitted from the screen is simultaneously suppressing your melatonin release and screwing with your circadian rhythm. Of course, few people appreciate the importance of circadian rhythms and the light-dark cycle because modern health research is instead preoccupied with the demonization of perfectly healthy foods like red meat and eggs and convincing as many healthy people as possible to embrace toxic statin drugs.

But I digress.

Industrialized populations are frequently exposed to higher levels of ambient air pollution. They eat foods laced with an endless list of chemical additives, the health effects of which are ultimately unknown. They consume alcohol and an endless list of recreational and prescription drugs, all of which can exert potent side effects.

Primitive populations are less likely to display high bodily iron stores, thanks to high levels of physical activity and also the ubiquity of parasitic infections that increase intestinal blood loss and hence iron loss. Iron is a potent pro-oxidant, and the FeAST study showed that reducing bodily iron stores, even in a half-assed manner, reduced the incidence of cancer [5].

Speaking of parasites, primitive populations tend to be marked by higher levels of infectious disease. They lack the sanitation and hygienic facilities and practices prevalent among industrialized populations. This is a major reason why average life expectancies in primitive populations are much lower than those seen in modernized nations. Populations that have lower life expectancies as a result of infectious disease will inevitably display patterns of chronic disease different to those of modernized populations for the simple fact microbes will kill many of them before chronic diseases do.

These are just some of the physiological factors that may explain variations in disease patterns, and we haven't even discussed psychosocial stressors yet. Primitive populations are focused on the day-to-day necessities of finding food, shelter, and in some instances protecting themselves from both human and wild animal predation. Their psychosocial stressors, therefore, tend to be of an acute short-term nature, unlike the stressors of modern life, which are ever present and create a constant, low level of adrenergic stimulation. Unlike modern folks, primitive peoples do not go into crippling debt to accumulate overpriced status symbols or put their kids through college, they don't endure lengthy and expensive divorce settlements, they don't grind away for years on end at jobs they hate, and they don't sit and fume in traffic jams.

I could go and on, but my point is that the ways in which industrialized and non-industrialized differ is almost endless.

And so there could have been many explanations for the difference in chronic disease patterns of industrialized versus developing countries. Despite this, Denis Parsons Burkitt honed in on and became thoroughly enamoured with a grand total of just *one*:

Fibre.

And hence we encounter another huge problem with epidemiology. It is a highly convenient tool for researchers who become single-mindedly infatuated with a particular health or dietary factor. Having embraced this factor, it is easy to construct a supportive case based on epidemiology. You gather up the data for a bunch of populations, compare the incidence of disease in those populations, note that your pet factor is *associated* with the incidence of disease among these populations, and triumphantly conclude this factor explains the increased prevalence of chronic disease in modernized populations. You largely or totally ignore the myriad of other possible factors, and you ignore the fact that any association between your pet factor and disease incidence is just that: Nothing more than a *statistical association*.

Which, of course, is exactly what Burkitt did.

The Diverticulitis Diversion

To get his hypothesis rolling, Burkitt used the example of diverticulitis (a.k.a. diverticulosis), a disease in which pouches form in the wall of the colon, often leading to inflammation and infection. In his seminal 1971 paper *"Diverticular Disease of the Colon: A Deficiency Disease of Western Civilization,"* Burkitt and his colleague Neil Painter noted the incidence of diverticulitis was much lower among rural Africans and Asians than among North American blacks, an observation Burkitt would repeatedly cite in his subsequent writings. Japanese people living in Hawaii, they also noted, had a higher incidence of this disorder than their cousins back home.

Burkitt blamed the advent of flour milling and the subsequent reduction in cereal fibre intake for the increased rates of diverticulitis in modernized societies. And so the whole-grain theory was launched in earnest [6]. This is an interesting point of distinction--health authorities could have chosen to emphasize vegetable fibre intake instead of cereal fibre, but the latter stole the limelight due to Burkitt's musings, and because cereal grains were the major staple in both industrialized and non-industrialized countries alike.

The bias towards cereal fibre ignored the fact that cereal grains were a relatively recent introduction to the human diet, unlike the fresh non-cereal vegetation that humans had been consuming for millions of years.

Burkitt believed his fibre theory also explained disparities in colorectal cancer rates:

"My interest in fiber as a possible protection against large bowel cancer was triggered by the observation that this form of cancer appeared to have a geographical distribution similar to that of diverticular disease. It was becoming apparent at that time, that this latter disorder was the result of a deficiency of fiber in the diet."[7]

As we saw earlier, there were a myriad of factors that could have contributed to the geographical co-existence of bowel cancer and diverticulitis, but Burkitt's fascination with faeces effectively blinkered him. He claimed:

"It is of interest that no community with high fecal output has anywhere been shown to have other than a low rate of colorectal cancer."

Burkitt wasn't all about the colon though. Hell no. He believed the protective effects of fibre extended to anatomical regions far beyond those related to the disposal of doo-doo.

"Breast cancer," he noted, *"occurs about eight times as frequently in black American women as in African women. Incidence rates rise when Japanese women immigrate to Hawaii. The factors responsible for these changes must be largely environmental. Breast cancer incidence is inversely related to age of menarche in various communities, and this in turn appears to be related to fiber intake. This could be due to the effect of fiber on*

the metabolism of cholesterol, which is a precursor of hormones that influence uterine development."[7]

Burkitt clearly believed his fibre theory explained a lot about modern disease patterns, but here was just one wee problem with his thesis: It was riddled with more holes than a bullet-ridden sieve.

The Evidence that Burkitt and his Followers Ignored

Burkitt made much ado about the difference in diverticulitis incidence among rural Africans and African-Americans, but the two populations lived starkly contrasting lifestyles on totally separate continents. A far more valid comparison would have been to compare rural and urbanized peoples in the same area of Africa, which is exactly what South African researchers Isidor Segal & Alexander Walker did.

The pair examined the dietary habits and incidence of diverticulitis among blacks in Soweto, most of whom had been urban dwellers for one or more generations. The traditional diet of their rural counterparts was low in fat and high in fibre; while the diet of urbanized blacks was still low in fat (24% of calories), their dietary fibre intake was very low (only 14 grams daily). Some of the dietary changes that contributed to this disparity were the adoption of refined maize as the staple cereal, decreased consumption of fruits and vegetables, and the increased consumption of animal protein, salt, and sugar--the very changes Burkitt believed to be behind the Western increase in diverticulitis.

Except that the urbanized blacks of Soweto, eating their low-fibre diets, enjoyed very low rates of diverticulitis, similar to those of their roughage-munching rural cousins![8]

Then there was Burkitt's repeated citation of native versus Hawaiian Japanese. The former, with their low rates of diverticulitis and breast cancer, were supposedly a shining demonstration of the value of cereal fibre.

This was a claim that flippantly ignored the fact that the primary source of calories in Japan was *white* rice. Asians had been refining their rice long before the advent of modern milling technology. While it takes a lot longer to mill rice by hand, Asians went to the trouble regardless because they believed (and not without foundation) that white rice was more digestible than brown, and that removing the husk also removed impurities and contaminants (as I'll discuss in Part II, the outer husk of rice acts as a magnet for arsenic)[9]. White rice also had the advantage of a much longer shelf life; when you've endured the labour-intensive process of harvesting your cereal crop by hand, you sure as heck want to make sure as little as possible is lost to spoilage.

Oh, and need I mention that white rice continues to dominate the diet of the Japanese, who still enjoy lower rates of breast and colorectal cancer than most Western countries?

One important factor that Burkitt did mention but quickly glossed over was the glaring discrepancy in longevity between rural Africans and residents of industrialized nations. The frequency of diverticulitis, like many chronic diseases, rises markedly as people age. Post-mortem studies estimate the prevalence to be 5%-10% of patients up to the age of 50, 50% of those over 60 years of age, and 66% of those over 85 years of age [10]. Given that the average life expectancy of rural Africans was (and still is) much lower than that of Western citizens, it's hardly surprising that diverticulitis was far more common in the West (average 1970 life expectancy in Uganda, for example, was only 49.9 years, and as of 2011 had improved marginally to 55.8 years[11]).

The Biggest Flaw of All

It's bad enough when researchers cherry-pick the epidemiological evidence that appears to support their thesis, but the biggest problem of all with Burkitt's fibre theory is that it was embraced and accepted as fact by health authorities *before* randomized clinical trials were conducted to test its veracity. These trials should have been conducted and analysed *before* health authorities began subjecting us to an endless stream of whole-grain propaganda, and *before* clueless book authors, journalists and other assorted health 'experts' began bombarding us with politically correct but scientifically untenable admonitions to eat more whole-grains.

But they didn't. When Burkitt's co-author, Neil Painter, published a paper in 1982 with the audacious title *"Diverticular disease of the colon. The first of the Western diseases shown to be due to a deficiency of dietary fibre"* [12], he should have been met with a flurry of criticism highlighting the fact that neither diverticulitis nor any other disease had ever been *"shown"* to be due to a *"deficiency"* of dietary fibre. But he wasn't. Instead, the pseudoscientific theory he crafted with Burkitt was accepted in dolt-like fashion, with virtually no objective and critical analysis, by the same unthinking mainstream that brought us the cholesterol theory of heart disease, the glorification of trans fat-laden margarines and linoleic acid-rich refined oils, and the pseudoscientific superstition against red meat. Some researchers did point out the flaws in Burkitt and Painter's hypothesis, but were largely ignored [13]. Never the type to learn from their mistakes, 'prestigious' health authorities, as well as the researchers, medical personnel, journalists, and popular book authors who blindly accepted their edicts, embraced yet another useless dietary theory with no foundation in sound science.

Which is yet another *massive* problem with modern-day dietary and health 'experts.' They have a hopeless obsession with data from epidemiological studies. They accept the statistical associations in these studies at face value, as if they were causal. Along with the pervasive and untoward influence of financially vested interests, the modern obsession with epidemiology is a major reason why modern dietary recommendations and primary prevention of chronic disease are of such appalling inefficacy.

Why Epidemiology is one of the Biggest Shams in Medical Science

Epidemiological studies can detect associations between dietary variables and disease incidence (we'll ignore for now that the strength of those associations is often pathetically weak), but they do *nothing* to explain *why* those associations exist.

I'll give you a quick hypothetical example to illustrate my point. Let's pretend you and I are researchers working for the Ministry of Statistical Chicanery, and one day the minister calls us into his office. He tells us the word on the street is that red motor vehicles are involved in a disproportionately high number of traffic accidents. He wants us to pull up all the traffic accident reports for the People's Republic of 'Straylia, crunch the numbers, and see if there is in fact a higher incidence of accidents involving red cars.

And so we trudge back to our computers, log off eBay, and get to work. We pull up all the stats for motor vehicle accidents, place them into separate categories according to the colour of the cars involved, and run the numbers to see if there is any correlation between vehicle colour and accident susceptibility.

Lo and behold, there is! When the data is tallied up, it shows unmistakably that the accident rate for red cars is double the average for all other colours combined. We print out our report, excitedly barge into the minister's office, and proudly relay our findings.

The minister is absolutely delighted with what he sees. *"Great work guys!"* he exclaims.

He then sits in deep, silent thought for a moment before triumphantly blurting out his solution to the problem:

"A national car-repainting program!"

"What?!"

"In order to cut the nation's road accident rate, the Ministry will issue an executive order that all red cars in 'Straylia have to be repainted another colour by December 31! And starting from the same date, the production and import of all red cars will be prohibited in 'Straylia!"

"Boss..."

"Yes Anthony?"

"That's a crap idea."

"What?!"

"It's a crap idea, a complete load of horseshit. For starters, all we've done is detect a statistical association between red cars and increased accident frequency. This tells us nothing about what is actually causing this relationship. Your solution assumes that the red duco itself is a causal factor, but there are a myriad of other factors that could be involved."

"Like what, wise guy?"

"Well, our data show that owners of red cars tend to be younger and have less driving experience. That right there could explain much of the disparity in accident rates. However, when we ran our highly sophisticated Multivariate Linear Cox Regression Correlate Coefficient Multiple Shoop Shoop Diddy Wop Rama Lama Ding Dang Analysis to account for age and

driving experience, the association with red duco and increased accident susceptibility was slightly weakened but still remained statistically significant. This leads us to suspect that the kinds of people who prefer red vehicles may also exhibit other characteristics that predispose to higher accident susceptibility, such as greater impulsivity, exhibitionism and risk-taking, and greater aggression behind the wheel. But to confirm this suspicion we'd need to recruit a random sample of the driving population and conduct the appropriate interviews and tests."

"Go on..."

"If these interviews and tests did indeed reveal a riskier profile among red car drivers, then we'd have to conclude it's driver behaviour and not car duco itself that is causing the higher accident rate. Red cars don't kill people, people do! We would then know that the most effective strategy is to target driver behaviour, instead of instigating some useless nationwide wank that focuses on eliminating red cars. If you wanted to confirm the innocence of red paint conclusively, we could even conduct a trial in which we randomly assign some of the government's car fleet to be painted various colours, including red, and tally up the subsequent accident rate. I think you'll find the relationship between red cars and accidents will disappear because in this instance the cars are being chosen for the drivers, instead of the drivers choosing the cars."

"Goddamnit Colpo, always the voice of reason and common sense, aren't you? Can't you ever just keep the peace and go along with the Ministry's proposals?"

"No. Because your proposals are inherently stupid, focus on statistical red herrings instead of actual causes, and waste truckloads of taxpayer money on useless interventions. And in this instance, your proposal will ultimately result in unnecessary

loss of human life, because the accident rate will remain unaffected while you jokers bark up the wrong tree."

The hypothetical scenario I've presented above pretty much encapsulates the history of modern nutritional epidemiology. Findings that did nothing more than relay statistical associations of unknown cause and veracity have been widely accepted as physiological fact, which in turn has led to the formation of patently false theories and the widespread embrace of diet and health interventions--sometimes on a global scale--that have proved utterly useless.

Again, one of the major reasons modern primary prevention of heart disease and cancer has been such a monumental failure, as reflected by the fact that incident rates of these diseases have remained virtually unchanged despite years of anti-fat, anti-cholesterol, anti-red meat and pro-whole-grain propaganda, is because of the modern infatuation with epidemiology.

Combined with the accompanying wanton disregard for controlled clinical trial findings that fail to support such untenable and prematurely-embraced theories, the result has been almost total impotence by health authorities in their primary prevention efforts against chronic diseases such as CVD, cancer, and diabetes.

The Correct Way to Test a Theory

If we detect an association between cereal fibre and diverticulitis in a nutritional epidemiological study, we have no right to proclaim that association as causal until we have tested it under controlled circumstances.

We need to conduct what is known as a randomized controlled clinical trial (RCT).

This is where we recruit as many subjects as our budget will allow, and randomly split them into two groups. Both groups will be assigned to follow similar diets, except that one group will consume a higher amount of fibre. This gives us a huge advantage over epidemiological studies, because by randomly assigning subjects to their diets helps eliminate a vast array of potential confounding factors. Scores of epidemiological studies, for example, have claimed harmful effects for red meat consumption, but when we look at the baseline characteristics of the study participants, the red meat eaters invariably display lower rates of physical activity, higher rates of smoking, alcohol consumption, and overweight, and even poorer sleep habits. Little wonder that these subjects often suffer worse health outcomes, but the researchers responsible for these studies routinely go ahead and blame red meat consumption any old how.

Randomization, in contrast, helps ensure that both groups in a trial have a similar mean age, similar numbers of smokers, similar exercise habits, similar proportion of males and females, and so on. Randomization eliminates the phenomenon of health-conscious trial participants self-selecting themselves for the diet or intervention that is, rightly or wrongly, perceived as healthier by authorities and the general public.

Along with recruiting the desired number of participants, we will set a time span for the trial, one that from previous observation should be long enough for susceptible subjects to develop diverticulosis symptoms. During that time period we will tally up the number of people who are diagnosed with diverticulosis. We will also record the incidence of other adverse health effects, and also record any deaths that occur in either group during the study period. This is important, because any observed reduction in diverticulosis will be little cause for celebration if there is a higher rate of other adverse health effects or deaths in the fibre group.

If, at the end of the study, we observe no reduction in diverticulosis rates among subjects assigned to eat more fibre, then we have strong grounds for assuming that the fibre theory is highly suspect. If subsequent high quality trials by other researchers also fail to find any benefit for high fibre diets, then we can pretty much assume that the theory is a load of bollocks.

Well, guess what? A number of such trials have already been performed, but their results are largely ignored by those enamoured with the fibre theory. Let's find out why.

Burkitt's Diverticulitis Theory on Trial

Between 1972 and 1985, several *non-randomized* trials compared the effect of fibre supplementation on diverticulitis [14-18]. All four studies reported a reduction in diverticulitis symptoms, and some also claimed a reduced need for surgery in the fibre groups. But these studies were inherently flawed by the same problem plaguing epidemiological studies--lack of randomization and hence an inability to control for confounding factors. One study, for example, reported that 91% of patients remained asymptomatic during 5-7 years' follow-up, however, only 75% adhered to a high-fibre diet, indicating that placebo effect may have been at least partially responsible for the difference [17].

Weight loss may also have been a confounding factor in at least one of these studies. Brodribb et al briefly mentioned weight loss occurred after bran consumption (mean bodyweight 69.4 kg before, 68 kg after), but promptly dismissed the difference as insignificant and gave the matter no further discussion. Since this 1976 paper, however, abundant research has been published showing even small bodyweight losses can produce significant improvements in many health markers, including glycaemic control. Brodribb et al's data actually support these subsequent findings; they observed an improvement (reduction) in the blood glucose response to an oral glucose tolerance test, one that could not be explained by the widely-held belief that cereal fibre slows carbohydrate release into the bloodstream. As the researchers admitted: *"This does not seem to have been due to a change in gastric emptying, as the rate of rise at 30 minutes was comparable. Fibre in food can increase the rate of transit through the small intestine, but the patients had not taken bran for at least 12 hours before the glucose tolerance test was carried out."*[16]

Only one of these non-randomized studies (Leahy et al 1985) reported deaths during the trial, and the results are disconcerting, to say the least. While relief of diverticulitis symptoms was reportedly greater among those who consumed 25 grams or more of fibre daily, 23% of the high-fibre subjects died during the study compared to only 8% of the low-fibre subjects. This disparity occurred despite a much longer mean follow-up period for the latter (54 versus 76 months, respectively)[18]. The researchers wrote: *"none of these deaths was related to diverticular disease or its complications,"* but no details about the actual causes of these deaths were given. And even if the deaths were unrelated to diverticulitis, that doesn't mean they were unrelated to fibre--as you'll learn in Part II, higher rates of adverse health effects and even death are not the exception in clinical trials involving increased cereal fibre intake, *but the norm.*

One of the above research groups dropped the non-randomization gig and subsequently proceeded with a double-blind RCT of patients with symptomatic diverticular disease. The results, published in 1977, were far from inspiring. The study involved only 18 patients who were randomly allocated either to a wheat crisp bread supplying 0.6 g of fibre daily or a bran crisp bread containing 6.7 g of fibre daily. The patients were followed for three months and interviewed monthly to determine compliance and to complete the enrolment questionnaire again.

It's important to note that in this study the determination of symptoms relied entirely upon questionnaires; no clinical examination or testing was employed at any point during the study. Hence, the results were susceptible to the vagaries of subjective recall and memory. This method of determining self-reported symptoms returned a highly significant reduction in the mean overall symptom score for the nine patients in the high-fibre group compared to controls. But although the high-fibre group experienced a significant decline in the pain score, there were no significant differences in the dyspeptic and bowel dysfunction scores [19].

Another RCT was reported this same year, but only ever published in abstract form. The study involved eighty diverticulosis patients randomized to one of 6 treatments: high-fibre, low-fibre, or no specific diet, or the aforementioned diets plus Metamucil or placebo. No significant differences were noted between the high- and low-fibre diets. Only Metamucil supplementation produced a significant reduction of symptoms and more patients without symptoms, although (again) no radiological confirmation of these findings was mentioned [20].

There was one more RCT whose results were published in 1977. In this study, thirty patients with diverticular disease confirmed by barium enema examination were entered into a 3-month double-blind trial comparing 2 x 500mg tablets of methylcellulose or 2 placebo tablets daily. The tablets were indistinguishable, allowing the researchers to cross over nine subjects and follow them for a further 3-month period.

It should be noted that methylcellulose does not occur in nature, but is chemically derived from cellulose (in this instance, from cotton or wood). The placebo effect was sufficient for eleven patients who completed the trial on placebo to show a small mean improvement. A greater mean clinical improvement was shown, however, by the sixteen patients who completed the trial on methylcellulose, leading some to conclude that the latter produced superior results. However, the mean reductions in symptom score among the placebo and methylcellulose subjects were 4.7 and 6.0, respectively--a piddling difference of 1.3 that was not statistically significant. The researchers also noted that nine of the patients participated in a further crossover study in which they spent three months each on placebo and methylcellulose. The greatest improvement was seen in the first three months where six of the nine subjects were taking methylcellulose, which the researchers took as further evidence of the possible superiority of methylcellulose [21].

In reality, the study proves nothing of the sort; two of the three patients who took the placebo during the first three-month phase did in fact also experience improvements. All we do know for sure is that the study was conducted in less-than-optimal fashion. For the crossover portion of the study, equal numbers of patients should have been assigned to two groups, one of which was administered the placebo during the first three months and the other methylcellulose, before swapping over for the last three months.

The results of the next RCT were published in 1981. This was a double-blind endeavour involving fifty-eight patients with symptomatic diverticular disease and lasting four months. The entire study was conducted in crossover fashion, which meant all subjects spent equal periods on both the fibre and placebo treatments. Two forms of dietary fibre supplement and two placebos were compared. The active treatments were bran biscuits (supplying 6.99 grams of fibre daily) and a drink made from powdered ispaghula husk (fibre 9.04 g/daily), while the placebos were crisp bread and a placebo powder both prepared from refined wheat (2.34 g/daily).

Importantly, assessments were made not just subjectively--using a monthly self-administered questionnaire--but also objectively, by examining a seven-day stool collection at the end of each treatment period.

In terms of pain score, lower bowel symptom score (incomplete emptying, straining, stool consistency, flatulence, and laxatives taken), and total symptom score (belching, nausea, vomiting, dyspepsia, and abdominal distension), fibre supplementation conferred no benefit.

The only symptom showing improvement was a reduction in constipation. While not an unworthy outcome, it clearly had little effect on diverticulitis, leading the researchers to conclude *"that dietary fibre supplements in the commonly used doses do no more than relieve constipation. Perhaps the impression that fibre helps diverticular disease is simply a manifestation of Western civilisation's obsession with the need for regular frequent defecation."*[22]

That damn doo-doo obsession again...

The bottom line is that high-quality evidence showing that cereal fibre benefits diverticulitis patients is essentially non-existent. And, thankfully, more independent-thinking researchers are stepping forward to point this out. As a group of Dutch researchers concluded in a recent review of the subject, authorities continue to recommend increased fibre for diverticulitis patients even though *"High-quality evidence for a high-fibre diet in the treatment of diverticular disease is lacking, and most recommendations are based on inconsistent level 2 and mostly level 3 evidence"* (i.e., evidence of poor quality)[23].

When Singaporean gastroenterologists Choon Sheong Seow and Francis Seow-Choen reviewed the evidence, they came to similar conclusions:

"There is sparse clinical evidence to support the widespread use of dietary fibre to alleviate abdominal symptoms or to prevent complications in uncomplicated diverticulosis. We provide a perspective contrary to conventional wisdom, and believe that a high-fibre diet confers little or no benefit and may even exacerbate the abdominal symptoms in these patients and increase the risks of diverticulitis or complications. More evidence in the form of long-term interventional study coupled with a group on high fibre and a control group without any fibre at all is needed before dietary fibre can be recommended for the treatment of diverticular disease."[24]

It's worth mentioning at this point another intestinal ailment that can cause its sufferers much grief--Irritable Bowel Syndrome (IBS). As with diverticulitis, increased fibre intake and/or fibre supplementation has long been recommended to IBS patients, but RCTs have repeatedly shown this strategy to be an overwhelming flop. In fact, increased cereal fibre intake has been shown in some trials to make the condition *worse* [25]. And never underestimate the power of placebo. In one telling double-blind RCT,

IBS patients received either three biscuits daily each containing ten grams of bran or regular wheat biscuits of similar appearance for six weeks. 52% of the patients in the treatment group reported *subjective* improvement of symptoms, which sounds great…until you read further and learn that 65% of the control group receiving the low-fibre placebo reported similar improvements![26]

Now You See it, Now You Don't

Before wrapping up Part I of our whole-grain myth dissection, I'd like to highlight something else about epidemiology. It routinely contradicts itself. But true to form, biased researchers and health authorities continue to select the epidemiological studies that support their own theories and ignore those that don't.

A couple of studies illustrating that point were recently published by a team of researchers from the University of North Carolina School of Medicine and the Albert Einstein College of Medicine, New York. They noted, *"Many physicians and patients believe that a high-fiber diet and frequent bowel movements prevent the development of diverticulosis. Evidence for these associations is poor."*

And so they recruited over 2,000 patients undergoing an outpatient colonoscopy at the University of North Carolina Hospitals in Chapel Hill, North Carolina. The patients, aged between 30 and 80, were given questionnaires about their usual dietary intake and physical activity levels. They were also divided into *"cases"* and *"controls"* based on their colonoscopy results;

cases (n = 878) were the patients found to have diverticula, controls (1,226) were those without diverticula noted on their colonoscopy report.

So what did the researchers find?

Patients with diverticulosis were more likely to be older, white, overweight or obese, to use tobacco, and to take non-steroidal anti-inflammatory drugs (NSAIDS) compared to those without diverticula.

And fibre intake? The raw data showed a trend towards increased diverticulitis with *higher* fibre intakes. When the data was mathematically adjusted in an attempt to account for potential confounders, this trend became clear, consistent, and statistically significant. As intake of total fibre, fibre from cereal grains, insoluble fibre, and soluble fibre increased, so too did the likelihood of being diagnosed with diverticulitis. Fibre from fruits and vegetables and beans showed no statistically significant relationship with diverticulitis diagnosis, nor did red meat or total fat intake. The initial inverse relationship between physical activity and diverticulitis disappeared after adjustment.

Oh, and constipation was not associated with a higher prevalence of diverticulosis. Instead, compared to individuals with less frequent (<7) bowel movements per week, those having 7 bowel movements had a higher prevalence (relative risk increase = 34%), as did those with 8–14 bowel movements per week (RR = 59%), and >15 bowel movements per week (RR = 70%) after adjustment for potential confounders [27].

That folks, pretty much refutes everything claimed by Burkitt and his extremely selective epidemiology.

Interestingly, the disparity between cereal fibre and fibre from fruits and vegetables was also seen in another epidemiological study examining diet and diverticulitis risk. As part of the Health Professionals Follow-up Study, 51,529 male health professionals without a history of diagnosed diverticular disease were followed for up to 4 years. Only 385 cases of symptomatic diverticular disease were diagnosed during this period, and an inverse association with high-fibre intake was observed. However, further analysis showed that while fruit and vegetable intake, cellulose, hemicellulose, and lignin were inversely associated with risk of symptomatic diverticular disease, cereal fibre was not [28].

Concluding Part I

Many of you reading this may have fallen for the mainstream claim that increased whole-grain intake imparts a plethora of health benefits. The purpose of Part I was to trace the origins of this claim, and to highlight its dubious nature. The thesis was formed by a researcher who harboured what some would consider a rather odd fascination with human faeces. This fascination led him to believe that the size and consistency of a person's stools were significant predictors of diverticulitis incidence and chronic disease susceptibility. He supported his belief with selectively cited epidemiological evidence, and he downplayed or flatly ignored the many blatant contradictions to his theory.

When controlled clinical trials examining the diverticulitis issue were finally conducted, they failed to confirm the fibre theory. Subsequent epidemiological studies have also failed to support the relationship between high cereal fibre intakes and reduced diverticulitis risk claimed by Burkitt and others.

Needless to say, this is not a particularly sound foundation for a theory that has come to dominate modern dietary beliefs.

These beliefs include the widely-accepted tenets that replacing refined grains with whole-grains will improve blood sugar control and reduce your risk of heart disease and cancer. In Part II, we'll examine the abundant clinical evidence showing that not only do whole-grains confer no such protection, but are in fact more likely to *increase* your risk of these health problems.

Part II

"Today, the Junksters believe that statistics are science and that statistical correlations represent cause-and-effect relationships. Wrong again."
Steve Milloy, *Junk Science Judo*

Ladies and gentlemen, welcome to Part II of my dissection of the whole-grain myth. This myth would have you believe that all sorts of awesome health benefits await if only you'd swap your white bread for brown and start eating brown rice instead of white.

While politically correct, this claim is scientifically very incorrect. In fact, it's complete rubbish.

In Part I, we traced the origins of the fantasy-based whole-grain cereal hypothesis. It began in the early 70s when Denis Burkitt, a UK researcher with a rather odd fascination for human faeces, claimed that a lack of cereal fibre caused diverticulitis. He promptly expanded his theory to include fibre 'deficiency' as a cause of other chronic diseases such as colorectal and breast cancers.

As explained in Part I, Burkitt formed his hypothesis, not by anything resembling thorough scientific scrutiny, but by a mix of creative thinking and evasion of contradictory evidence. Nevertheless, thanks to his prior and admirable achievements as a missionary in Africa and the appalling lack of scientific rigor so regrettably pervasive among our 'health authorities', Burkitt's claims were readily accepted as fact. It's now over forty years since Burkitt first published his theory, and there is still no controlled evidence to support the cereal fibre thesis. Yet health organizations, researchers, book authors, journalists, dieticians, and scores of others who pretend to know something worthwhile about nutrition stubbornly persist in claiming whole-grains are good for us.

Industry-Funded Fantasy

Among the purported goals of the Whole Grain Council (WGC), a group formed by *"concerned millers, manufacturers, scientists and chefs,"* are to help *"consumers find whole grain foods and understand their health benefits,"* and help *"the media write accurate, compelling stories about whole grains."* According to the WGC, whole-grains lower the risk of heart disease, stroke, diabetes, obesity, asthma, colorectal cancer, high blood pressure…even gum disease and tooth loss!

To see what kind of evidence they rely upon to arrive at these conclusions, you can visit their website and freely download a number of summaries. Clicking on the WGC Research Summary (http://wholegrainscouncil.org/files/WGResearchSummary_WGCJan09.pdf) and perusing the studies they've cited is most instructional. And rather amusing or depressing, depending on your individual predisposition. It lists *"almost four dozen studies,"* most of which supposedly demonstrate the wonderful health benefits of whole grain cereals. But take a good look at the type of studies listed. The overwhelming majority are epidemiological studies (these are the ones marked *"prospective," "case control,"* or *"cross-sectional"*).

Dietary epidemiological studies, as you learned in Part I, are largely a load of overrated, confounder-prone hogwash. If you think I'm being harsh, I'm not. It's hard to fathom the amount of unnecessary human misery caused by the modern obsession with epidemiology and the stunningly stupid habit of holding the results of these studies in the same regard as clinical trial data. If you have a loved one that died of heart disease, cancer, or diabetes complications in the last few decades, imagine what their prognosis may have been if modern medicine committed itself to hunting down the real culprits instead of wasting billions of dollars and incalculable manpower on the misleading statistical chicanery that characterizes modern nutritional epidemiology. It's the same chicanery, I should note, that brought us such utterly useless and often counterproductive pseudoscientific wankery as cholesterol reduction, saturated fat restriction, red meat avoidance, and high cereal fibre intakes.

Nutritional epidemiological studies are capable of detecting nothing other than statistical associations of unknown cause. To get any kind of reliable insight as to whether the association between, say, higher self-reported whole-grain intakes and lower risk of disease is causal, we need to conduct a randomized controlled clinical trial (RCT). This allows us to largely remove the possible effect of unforeseen confounding factors that would otherwise sway the results of non-randomized and totally uncontrolled epidemiological studies.

Keeping that in mind, let's return to the WGC's Research Summary. If you look at the small number of clinical trials they've cited (Table 3), you'll notice they're all short-term endeavours examining changes in so-called *"risk factors"* such as serum cholesterol, blood glucose and insulin, CRP, and fructosamine.

There are a number of small--okay, majorly whopping--problems with the citation of these studies. First of all, some of them don't even compare refined grains with their whole-grain equivalents. One study, for example, compared the 2-hour post-meal effects of fermented whole-grain barley and oats with... pure glucose. In a world-shattering revelation, the fermented grains caused lower insulin and glucose responses than the purified glucose.

Another study compared a low-calorie diet containing whole grain *"double-fermented"* wheat with a diet containing... Slimfast.

No, I'm not kidding. It's right there in Table 3.

Another examines the effect of corn versus oat cereal on total and LDL cholesterol. Let's forget for a moment that the cholesterol theory of heart disease is quite possibly the finest example of authority-endorsed pseudoscientific stupidity in recent human history. Even if it had merit, why cite a study that compared two totally different cereals in support of the whole-grain hypothesis? Remember, we're trying to remove all possible confounders, so if you want to prove the whole version of a grain is superior, then you compare whole wheat with refined wheat, brown rice with refined rice, and so on.

But this is all small stuff compared to the major flaw of the trials cited in Table 3. The real problem is that not a single one of them examined actual disease incidence or mortality. And how could they, given that the longest one lasted a mere three months?

Wait a minute ... maybe the WGC folks saved the long-term clinical trials for Table 4, which lists *"studies comparing dietary patterns with morbidity and mortality"*?

Nope ... not a single RCT to be found. Table 4 is just more epidemihogwash.

Hmmm.

There have indeed been longer-term RCTs comparing refined and whole-grains, so why didn't the WGC list them in their *"Research Summary"*? I don't know about you, but I don't even begin to consider short-term changes in serum *"blood lipids"* and *"fructosamine"* levels a worthwhile reason to make fundamental changes to my dietary habits. Especially when those changes tend to taste like cardboard. I want some kind of hard evidence that such dietary modification might actually lower my risk of chronic disease or mortality.

Before we examine just why an organization devoted to the dissemination of pro-whole-grain material might be reluctant to cite the most important studies of all, let's take a look at the other papers they present in support of eating sawdust ... uh, I mean, whole-grains.

The next paper, which the WGC incorrectly lists as a *"meta-analysis,"* is in fact a summary of an American Society for Nutrition 2010 Symposium called *"Putting the Whole Grain Puzzle Together: Health Benefits Associated with Whole Grains."* As we proceed to discuss this summary, keep in mind one of the researchers responsible was an employee of General Mills, while three others had received funding from the company. General Mills, in fact, sponsored the entire symposium.

In this summary, the researchers conclude: *"There is consistent epidemiological evidence that whole grain foods substantially lower the risk of chronic diseases such as CHD, diabetes, and cancer and also play a role in body weight management and digestive health."*

Yeah, no kidding, we know about the dodgey epidemiology already. Where's the far more reliable long-term RCT data?

Well, as with the WGC, the authors of the ASN summary are, for some strange reason, reluctant to show it to us.

Despite completely failing to discuss this RCT data, they further claim in their conclusion that:

"Current evidence lends credence to the recommendations to incorporate whole grain foods into a healthy diet and lifestyle program."

The most ridiculous statement in the entire paper comes from one of the authors, Dr. Chris Seal of Newcastle University, Newcastle upon Tyne, who in the last two sentences of the paper is quoted as saying:

"Soon, only the ill-informed will avoid whole grains foods. Whole grains are not a luxury, and no house is complete unless they are provided at every meal."

Lawdy, lawdy…

Look, no disrespect to Dr. Seal, but that statement is not just false but patently ludicrous. As you will soon learn, only the ill-informed believe that whole-grain cereals offer tangible health benefits, and those who truly care about their health will avoid them as much as possible until folks like Dr. Seal can provide tightly-controlled evidence actually demonstrating these alleged health benefits.

So far, that evidence is completely lacking, which I guess is why it didn't feature in the ASN paper. Instead, we are subjected to the usual intelligence-insulting epidemiology, along with a meagre sprinkling of trials again examining only short-term changes in 'risk markers,' the long-term relevance of which is unknown.

Two Down, One to Go

The third paper linked to by the WGC, which they also incorrectly call a meta-analysis, is a review by a University of Minnesota professor who *"reviewed and compiled scores of recent studies on whole grains and health, to show how whole-grain intake is protective against cancer, cardiovascular disease, diabetes and obesity."*

You don't need me to tell you the rest, right?

Yep, more sloppy epidemiology and more largely irrelevant short-term clinical trials.

The author of this review is also a keen practitioner of the piecemeal "Irrelevant Extrapolation" approach to evidence acquisition. This is where you take several pieces of unrelated evidence with a common thread, and then place them together to make it look like you have a sound argument. One shining example is when she attempts to find mechanisms for the allegedly *"protective effects of whole grains"* against cancer. She cites phytic acid (a.k.a phytate, inositol hexaphosphate, IP6), noting that this iron-lowering substance has been shown to reduce cancer incidence in animals. It certainly has, but what the author fails to mention is that these studies invariably used, not phytate from whole-grains, but purified inositol hexaphosphate in the rodents' drinking water[29-34] In the one study that did also include cereal fibre, a diet comprised of 20% Kellogg's All Bran could only muster a statistically non-significant 11.4% reduction in tumour incidence. However, rats given 0.4% IP6 in drinking water, equivalent to that in the 20% All Bran diet, were 34% less likely to develop tumours. The total number of tumours was reduced by 49% in the IP6 group, and only 10% of the IP6 rats developed three or more tumours compared to 32% in the 20% bran diet[34].

A couple of lines from this paper remind me of the old Churchill quote about people who occasionally stumble over the truth, but then *"pick themselves up and hurry off as if nothing ever happened."* One of these is in the abstract, where the author writes:

"Although it is difficult to separate the protective properties of whole grains from dietary fibre and other components, the disease protection seen from whole grains in prospective epidemiological studies far exceeds the protection from isolated nutrients and phytochemicals in whole grains."

That's because *"the disease protection seen from whole grains in prospective epidemiological studies"* has absolutely nothing to do with whole-grains, and everything to do with the fact that whole-grain eaters are much more likely to be health-conscious people, and therefore significantly more likely to engage in a variety of other behaviours that actually do benefit health. A classic example of this phenomenon, which you can access freely <u>right here</u>, is the Iowa Women's Health Study. It is another General Mills-instigated project which, of course this review, the WGC, and the authors of the ASN paper all cite in support of their arguments. The Iowa study allegedly showed that whole-grain intake reduced CHD risk, but a quick look at the baseline data reveals the real reason behind this association. As whole-grain intake went up, so too did physical activity levels and the use of vitamin supplements. Smoking, meanwhile, declined significantly; while 25% of those in the lowest quintile of whole-grain intake were smokers, only 12% of those in the highest quintile sucked on artery-clogging cancer sticks [35]. Unlike whole-grains, exercise and smoking cessation exert real and clinically-demonstrated improvements in cardiovascular mortality and morbidity. These are the real reasons that whole-grain eaters in the Iowa and similar studies show lower risks of disease.

Epidemiologists, of course, will object by claiming they *"adjust"* for such confounders. This is the eminently laughable notion that, by employing mathematical formulas, epidemiologists suddenly become equipped with God-like powers that allow them to remove the confounding effects of exercise, smoking, education, BMI, etcetera after the fact.

Yep, just like that.

They can't of course. But that doesn't stop them from persisting in this absurd emperor-has-no-clothes charade in which they present their adjusted figures and expect us to believe that running a multivariate analysis formula on their computers magically confers the same confounder-removing effects as clinical randomization.

Note to epidemiologists: Get off the drugs, for crying out loud! You cannot properly and fully account for potential confounders by waving around a "statistical wand," no matter how fancy or pretty it looks. You need to remove them before the study even gets rolling. You know, like randomized clinical trials do. By randomly assigning people to whole- and refined-grain diets in a trial, you remove the self-selection effect seen in epidemiological studies in which those with healthier lifestyles also eat more whole-grains because the fluffy health magazines they read tell them to.

And when this self-selection effect is removed courtesy of randomization, whole-grains invariably fail to demonstrate any of the health benefits claimed for them in epidemiological studies.

Which brings us to another ironic quote from the Minnesota paper. Discussing the epidemiological association between whole-grain consumption and type 2 diabetes risk, the author correctly notes:

"These studies cannot provide direct causal proof of the effects of whole grains in lowering the risk of type 2 DM since confounding remains an alternative explanation in non-randomised settings."

However, both before and after this brief flirtation with common sense, the author continually talks about the *"protective"* effects of whole-grains, and goes on to state *"based on epidemiological studies and biologically plausible mechanisms, the scientific evidence shows that the regular consumption of wholegrain foods provides health benefits in terms of reduced rates of CHD and several forms of cancer."*

They do no such thing.

And that, ladies and gentlemen, is pretty much the state of the art when it comes to mainstream 'scientific' discussion of the whole-grain paradigm: a heavy reliance on confounder-prone epidemiology, a brief nod to only the short-term clinical trials, and complete evasion of the longer-term trials that actually tell us something about the effects of cereal fibre and whole-grains on real world disease and mortality outcomes.

In short, the whole thing is simply an evasive, self-serving exercise in junk science.

Well folks, propaganda time is over. It's time to look at the evidence that the whole-grain shills never tell you about.

Anti-Nutrients: They're Real, Nasty, & Right There in Your Whole-Grain Bread

Throughout evolution, the various species that make up the plant and animal kingdom have developed a wide array of defence mechanisms to ensure their continued survival. Unlike animals, plants cannot bite, claw, or run away when faced with danger, so they've instead evolved a variety of toxic compounds, known as anti-nutrients, which can cause adverse health effects in those who attempt to consume them[36,37,]. Because of their abundant anti-nutrient content, grains (along with beans and potatoes) are all inedible in their uncooked state, a fact that only the most audacious whole-grain cheerleader would attempt to deny. Eating these foods raw can result in severe, and sometimes fatal, illness. Sufficient cooking, of course, renders the above foods edible but only partially destroys the anti-nutrients they contain.

Before I explain just how this relates to our whole-grain dissection, let's take a look at the three main components of a grain kernel:

1. **Endosperm:** This inner component constitutes the bulk of the kernel and is mostly starch. Although it's what you are ingesting when you eat products made from refined flours, I'm guessing the term "white bread" is much more marketable, especially to heterosexual male consumers. I mean, would you buy *"SpermFresh™ 100% Endosperm Bread"*? Yeah, me neither.

2. **Germ:** Also found inside the kernel, this is the nutrient-rich embryo that will sprout and grow into a new plant.
3. **Bran:** This is the hard, dark, outer husk that encases and protects the above two components. It's also the part of the grain that health authorities want you to believe confers all manner of wonderful health benefits. It is high in fibre and contains a number of vitamins and minerals. Because a primary function of bran is to protect the inner contents of the kernel, it is also rich in anti-nutrients.

Bloating, Farting, Indigestion and Mineral Excretion are Good for You!

Perhaps the most common improvement people report upon banishing whole-grains from their diet is alleviation of the numerous gastrointestinal symptoms that previously plagued them, such as flatulence, burping, indigestion, stomach bloating, and symptoms indicative of excess gut permeability (a.k.a. leaky gut syndrome). It's interesting how the pro-whole-grain crowd either pretend these symptoms don't exist (despite being documented in clinical trials) or simply fob them off as no big deal. I've actually seen pro-fibre health commentators dismiss symptoms such as increased flatulence as *"harmless"* and insignificant. I'm guessing these are the same folks who break into hysterical laughter when their partner drops a nasty one on the couch.

For those of us whose sense of humour did progress beyond junior high, an examination of the various anti-nutrients found in cereals and their gastrointestinal effects is most instructive.

Enzyme Inhibitors

Fruit doesn't mind being eaten. But it doesn't like its seeds to be chewed and digested, because it needs them for future replication. And so one of the mechanisms used by fruit to ensure the continued propagation of its seeds is bitterness. The instinctive desire to spit out fruit seeds after inadvertently biting into them is nature's way of ensuring a mutually beneficial transaction for both consumer and consumed; the former obtains calories and vital nutrients from the highly nutritious flesh of the fruit, while the seed is expelled and returned to the soil where it will eventually sprout and grow into a whole new plant. In some plants, such as raspberries, the seeds are so small they frequently escape the crushing action of teeth, passing through the digestive system intact and subsequently being delivered to the soil when the consumer defecates.

Grains, on the other hand, don't want to be eaten. Not wanting to get all *"Wheat Belly"* on you, but it's true. And so they didn't evolve with a sweet, moist, eye-catchingly bright exterior with a few seeds inside; they evolved with their carbohydrate-rich kernels totally encased in a hard, inedible outer layer of bran. It's the plant equivalent of putting up a six-foot fence with a sign reading "BEWARE OF THE DOG," and for millions of years-- up until some 10,000 years ago-- humans got the message.

Grains line this outer wall with enzyme inhibitors to bind up predators' digestive enzymes. These ensure that enzymes within the seed responsible for initiating the sprouting process remain dormant until conditions are just right; that is, after the seed has been expelled back to the earth and has received sufficient nutrition to begin germinating.

But what does this mean to you, the human consumer, who has gone ahead and cooked and eaten the whole grain? Well, picture the digestive enzymes in your stomach, swimming through the gut to begin work on an incoming meal, doing what they're supposed to do, when all of a sudden they get jumped by masked enzyme inhibitors. These nasty-ass inhibitors, using the element of surprise, apply disabling Ju Jitsu holds on your digestive enzymes. Some inhibit alpha-amylase, an enzyme found mainly in saliva and pancreatic juices that breaks down starch and glycogen into glucose and maltose. Others get in the face of proteases which, as their name suggests, assist in the breakdown and digestion of protein. Your protease and alpha-amylase enzymes flail and wriggle around and try and break free, but to no avail. They can't do their job properly, your food doesn't get digested with full efficiency, and so you sit there bloated, gaseous, and blaming the dog for the embarrassing green cloud rapidly immersing your dining table.

Not a pretty picture.

Lectins

In addition to enzyme inhibitors, grains also contain lectins. These are carbohydrate-binding proteins with the ability to successfully bind to cell receptors intended for carbohydrate-containing molecules. As these receptors are found in virtually every cell of the body, lectins can bind to a remarkably wide range of organs and tissues, including your pancreas, muscles, mouth, stomach, intestines, kidney, skin, nervous system, reproductive organs, and blood [38]. Yep, these wandering little bastards can pretty much go anywhere.

Unlike most other anti-nutrients, lectins remain largely unaffected by cooking. They're also highly resistant to digestive breakdown and are thus able to survive in the gastrointestinal tract [39]. Lectins are very effective in increasing intestinal permeability, allowing for increased transport of both themselves and other uninvited guests across the gut wall into the bloodstream. Wheat lectin antibodies are frequently found in the blood serum of both normal and celiac individuals, and other human research shows that lectin from peanuts (which are in fact not a nut but a legume) appears in the bloodstream as soon as one hour after ingestion [40].

In rodent studies, wheat lectin has been shown to cause pancreatic enlargement, intestinal damage that interferes with digestive and immune function, and shrinkage of the thymus gland which, because of its role in producing t-lymphocytes that attack harmful foreign molecules in the body, is a crucial component of the immune system [41].

In the interests of non-dodgey extrapolation, I must point out that the levels of wheat lectin required to produce such effects in rats are substantially higher than those that would normally be encountered in the average human diet. No long-term studies have been conducted in humans examining the effects of chronic, low level wheat lectin consumption, but the results of a study involving moderate peanut consumption suggest that increased intake of lectin-rich foods could indeed have deleterious health consequences.

In this experiment, researchers tested colon tissue from 36 volunteers who had eaten 100 grams of peanuts daily for 5 days. In the 10 subjects displaying an antigen associated with colon and other cancers, known as the Thomsen-Friedenreich antigen, peanut ingestion caused a significant increase in colon cell division [42]. The implications are worrying, as accelerated cell division is a hallmark of tumour development. Keep this in mind when we take a look in a moment at the RCTs examining the effect of cereal fibre on colorectal adenoma and cancer incidence.

Phytin' to Hang on to Your Minerals

One of the sing-song arguments in favour of whole-grain consumption goes like this:
"Grains contain most of their nutrients in the outer layer, and when the grain is refined you lose all these nutrients and end up with an inferior product!"

This is a great example of how a half-truth gets blown into an oft-repeated piece of nutritional 'wisdom.' Grains do indeed contain most of their vitamins and minerals in their outer layers, but--hello--this is also where the anti-nutrients are hiding out!

Cereal grains contain abundant phosphorous in the form of the aforementioned inositol hexaphosphate, more commonly known as phytate. In the gastrointestinal tract, phytate binds with important minerals such as iron, calcium, magnesium, and zinc--effectively impairing their absorption and subsequent utilization by the body [43-45]. Attempting to improve one's mineral status by increasing whole-grain intake is, at best, a 'two-steps-forward, two-steps-backward' proposition. Substituting whole-grain for refined cereal grain products does indeed increase zinc, iron, and calcium intake, but also promptly increases the excretion of these nutrients so that overall mineral status either worsens or remains unchanged [45]. The last thing most people need is to impair the assimilation of such nutrients, many of which are already woefully inadequate in the average American diet [46-48].

High phytate intake is yet another factor believed to contribute to the high rate of bone disorders seen among developing populations who rely on unrefined grains for the bulk of their calories [49]. After observing increased mineral excretion in infants given bran preparations as a treatment for constipation, paediatric researchers warned that bran supplementation in this group should be approached with *"extreme caution"*[50].

The mineral content of whole-grains may be the subject of frequent praise by dieticians, but high phytate levels ensure that such acclaim is wholly undeserved. As professor Harold Sandstead, M.D., from the Department of Preventive Medicine & Community Health at the University of Texas Medical Branch, wrote;

"It appears that some health promoters who suggest that U.S. adults consume 30-35g of dietary fiber daily either have not done their homework or have simply ignored carefully done research on this topic. They appear to be unaware of the effects of phytate on mineral retention and the fact that many of the commonly consumed sources of fiber are rich in phytate..." [51]

And vitamins? Well, a substance known as pyridoxine glucoside, which has been shown to reduce the availability of vitamin B6 by 75-80%, occurs widely in plant foods, including cereal grains [52]. As a result, B6 from cereal grain products is absorbed with far less efficiency than that from animal foods [53]. Researchers who fed young men different foods containing pyridoxine glucoside found that as dietary glucoside levels increased, the vitamin B6 status of the subjects decreased [54]. Again, increased wheat fibre consumption merely worsens the situation. B6 from whole wheat bread is 5-10% less available than that from white bread, and the addition of wheat bran to the diets of young men reduced the availability of B6 by 17% [55,56].

Cereal grains not only contain no detectable vitamin D but also actively encourage deficiency of this important vitamin by impairing its absorption. It has long been recognized that high cereal grain consumption induces vitamin D deficiency in various animal species, including primates, our closest animal relatives [57,58,]. By studying the fate of radiolabeled vitamin D, researchers observed significantly increased excretion of vitamin D in healthy human volunteers fed 60 grams of wheat fibre daily [59].

Whole-grains are nutritious? Um, no they're not. So that's a brief look at some of the anti-nutrients found in whole-grains. The whole-grain shills will tell you that these anti-nutrients are no big deal, that cooking neutralizes them and renders them harmless, and therefore all is hunky dory.

The whole-grain shills, as you should have realized by now, are full of malarkey.

Whole-Grains on Trial

Awrighty folks, this is where we really get to the heart of the matter. I've kept noting how the whole-grain propagandists refuse to acknowledge the longer-term cereal fibre/whole-grain trials, but there's also a whole raft of important short-term trials they're not telling us about either. Let's check out the shorter-term trials first, then the longer-term projects.
The blatant lie that whole-grain feeding is 'healthy' was disproved long ago, and there is simply no excuse for supposedly 'educated' researchers to keep perpetuating it. As far back as 1949, researchers from the University of Ceylon in Colombo found feeding brown rice to healthy male medical students for three weeks worsened their calcium and magnesium status, even though their intakes of these nutrients were higher than

when they ate white rice. Three of the subjects were fed a brown rice diet for an extended period of 18 weeks, and their calcium and magnesium balances began to improve, suggesting an adaptation to their lowered absorption of these important minerals. That this adaptation was not sufficient was suggested by the data for week 19 of the experiment, when the reintroduction of white rice diet was accompanied by an immediate increase in the amounts of calcium and magnesium retained [60].

A 1960 paper by Indian researchers reported similar findings for calcium and warned *"the exclusive consumption of brown rice in diets containing marginal or submarginal amounts of calcium is not to be recommended as it may produce negative calcium balances."*[61]

A 1976 paper reported a tightly controlled metabolic ward study in Iran in which two men ate two different diets for 20 days each. During the first 20 days, more than 50% of their energy intake was provided by white bread. During the second 20-day period, the white bread was replaced with Bazari, a traditional whole grain bread. Apart from the different breads, the experimental diets contained identical amounts of cheese, milk, mutton, fruits and vegetables, beans, rice, turnips, oils, tea/water, and sugar.

Zinc balance was positive during the white bread diet but became negative during the Bazari period. Increased faecal excretion was responsible for the change. Calcium balance also declined in both men during the Bazari period, despite moderately increased calcium intakes. The high content of magnesium in the bread led to a nearly doubled intake during its consumption compared with white bread. However, magnesium excretion in faeces increased to a still greater extent while that in urine also rose substantially. Moderately negative magnesium balances resulted while Bazari was being consumed [62].

Japanese researchers fed low protein (0.5g/kg bodyweight) diets to healthy males--white rice was consumed for the first 14 days, then brown rice was eaten for the next 8 days. Not surprisingly, nitrogen balance was negative on both diets, but fell to a greater extent on the brown rice diet [63].

Anti-nutrients and their effects are very real, folks.

The Blood Sugar Sham

Another incessant claim for whole-grains is their supposedly lower glycemic index (GI) and hence diabetes-fighting effects.

In contrast to the official dogma, white and brown versions of the same rice variety return almost identical scores when subject to GI testing. The GI of white Doongara rice, for example, is 64; the corresponding score for brown Doongara rice is 66. Both versions also have virtually identical insulin index scores.

The GI of rice is largely determined by its amylose levels, not its fibre content. The varying amylose content of different rice varieties is why this grain shows such a wide range of scores on the GI charts, with high amylose varieties sporting significantly lower GI scores. Long grain rice strains have higher amylose contents than their short grain cousins, so wherever possible, opt for long-grain rices like Basmati and Doongara, as they tend to have lower GI scores than instant, converted, and short-grain varieties [64,65]. Jasmine is an exception to the rule as it sports a higher GI despite its long-grain status.

A recent clinical trial from China further puts lie to the claim that brown rice has some sort of anti-diabetic effect. Researchers randomly assigned 202 middle-aged adults with diabetes or a high risk for diabetes to consume either white or brown rice *ad libitum* for 16 weeks. No differences were noted in BMI, waist circumference, glycated hemoglobin, blood glucose, or insulin concentrations between the two groups [66].

And what about other grains?

With wheat and barley, the degree of milling does have an impact on the GI. A true "whole-grain" is one that hasn't been ground, but this would pose an impediment in terms of texture and palatability, so millers tend to employ varying degrees of processing with whole-grains. Products made from finely ground whole-grains-- more accurately referred to as wholemeal --might be much darker than their white equivalents, but their glycemic effects are virtually identical. Compared to wholemeal bread, bread made from 75% bulgur (cracked wheat) did produce a substantially lower GI, although the subsequent score of 69 hardly qualifies it as low-GI (even pure bulgur could only muster a GI score of 66). Barley fared better with a GI score of 39 for both 75% cracked barley bread and for whole barley itself [67].

Another study confirmed this effect in wheat- and maize-based products, but found the degree of processing did not have any significant effect on oat products; the latter returned low-GI values irrespective of whether they were in whole, rolled, or flour form. The reason for this is that oats contain an unusually high proportion of soluble viscous fibre that limits the rate of digestion [68].

Yet another study again found similar glycemic responses among white and finely-ground whole wheat and barley breads, but significantly lower blood glucose responses after ingestion of sourdough bread made from white flour (probably due to sourdough bread's higher organic acid content) [69].

By now you should be starting to see how the "eat-more-whole-grains-and-enjoy-lower-blood-sugar!" mantra of the whole-grain crowd is overly simplistic and rather poorly conceived. Nowhere in their abundant propaganda do they issue any caveat that GI-lowering effects may only be seen with cracked grain as opposed to wholemeal products. Perhaps due to issues with palatability, the former make up only a small percentage of commercially available whole-grain products, which of course limits the practical applicability of their low-GI whole-grain thesis. The whole-grain shills also tend to avoid discussion of the sourdough 'paradox'; the fact that sourdough white breads return significantly lower GI scores than fibre-rich wholemeal breads is an uncomfortable contradiction to their entire whole-grain, pro-fibre thesis.

So what kind of improvements in blood sugar control can we expect when commonly available whole-grain/wholemeal products are incorporated into people's diets?

The answer from clinical trials appears to be... bugger all.

In Europe, for example, researchers compared 146 individuals with metabolic syndrome who were randomized to a diet based on whole-grains or on refined cereal products for 12 weeks. The participants were aged 40-65 years and hailed from Kuopio, Finland and Naples, Italy. The participants were encouraged not to change their habitual meat, dairy product, egg, fish, fruit, vegetable and fat intake during the study; the only difference between the whole-grain and the control diet was the inclusion of a fixed amount of whole-grain (from whole wheat, rye, and oat products) or refined cereal products as the main carbohydrate source. The test products in both diets were provided free of charge to the participants in amounts sufficient to cover their household consumption for the whole duration of the study.

At the end of the study, there were no differences between the two groups in terms of weight change, blood pressure, triglycerides, blood glucose, or insulin levels. Mean levels of the latter three actually increased slightly on the whole-grain diet, but the changes were small and not statistically significant. Nevertheless, they hardly support the *ad nauseum* claim that whole-grains have some sort of anti-diabetic effect [70].

Swedish researchers conducted a similar experiment in crossover fashion, meaning that the subjects all spent six weeks on both whole-grain and refined cereal diets in random order. Again, no differences were noted in blood pressure, fasting blood glucose or insulin, or insulin sensitivity [71].

And what about all this talk we hear about whole-grains improving *"antioxidant protection"*? What exactly is being protected by supposedly *"antioxidant-rich"* whole-grains?

Nothing, basically. Whole-grains, for the record, are not antioxidant-rich foods nor do they boost antioxidant defences within the body.

When Jenkins et al gave type 2 diabetics a low-wheat fibre diet and a high-wheat fibre diet containing bran-rich bread and breakfast cereal for three months each, free radical damage of LDL cholesterol increased during the high-wheat fibre phase [72].

In a University of Minnesota experiment, healthy young males and females followed a refined grain diet or a diet in which refined grains were replaced by whole grain and whole meal products in random order. Despite its higher content of the antioxidant nutrients vitamin B6, folate, selenium, zinc, magnesium, and cysteine, the whole grain diet produced no improvement whatsoever in blood antioxidant capacity, nor in urinary markers of antioxidant status [73]. One of the authors of this study, Jennifer Slavin, was also the author of the third WGC-cited review I discussed earlier, and she's additionally written numerous other papers praising the protective 'antioxidant' effects of whole-grains. Yet her own clinical research confirms these mythical antioxidant effects don't exist.

Speaking of researchers whose own clinical experiments belie their hyperbolic claims about whole-grains, remember Dr. Chris Seal, the UK professor who claimed that *"Soon, only the ill-informed will avoid whole grains foods"*? Well, when he and a bunch of his fellow Newcastle University colleagues set out to confirm the 'heart healthy' effects of whole-grains, they came up short. In their own words:

"Although reported WG intake was significantly increased among intervention groups, and demonstrated good participant compliance, there were no significant differences in any markers of CVD risk between groups."

The subjects had been assigned to one of three groups: a control group or one of two intervention groups. Participants in intervention group 1 were asked to consume the equivalent of 60 grams of whole-grain daily (approximately equal to the whole-grain content of three slices of bread) for the whole 16-week period. Participants in intervention group 2 were asked to consume 60 grams of whole-grain daily for 8 weeks followed by 120 grams daily for the final 8 weeks. After 16 weeks, there were no differences between any of the groups in BMI, percentage body fat, waist circumference, glucose and insulin; nor were there any differences in indicators of inflammation, blood coagulation, and arterial function [74].

Like I said Dr. Seal, only the ill-informed believe that whole-grains offer health benefits.

In the abstract of their 2008 paper, Katcher et al reported reductions in CRP and abdominal fat in their whole-grain fed subjects, but neglected to mention that overall weight and fat loss was greater, albeit not statistically significantly, in the refined cereal group. What, if any, clinical significance the CRP change might represent should be considered in light of the fact that all other measures of inflammation and glycemic control were similar in both groups [75].

The Weight Loss Wank

Another oft-repeated claim is that refined grains make us fat while whole-grains, through some mystical, magical aberration of the laws of nature, help us lose weight.

What a crock. For the umpteenth time, an excess of calories is what makes people fat. It doesn't matter if that excess of calories comes from whole-grains or refined grains or pickled frog turd--if you eat beyond your caloric requirements for a sufficient length of time, then an excess of chub is the logical outcome. But hey, maybe the crap taste and inferior palatability of whole-grains results in some kind of spontaneous caloric reduction that in turn leads to weight loss?

Alas, this does not seem to happen.

As noted earlier, weight and fat loss was greater in Katcher et al's refined cereal group compared to their whole-grain group (-5.3 versus -3.7kg and -4.7% versus -2.5%, respectively).

When Bodinham et al assigned fourteen young healthy adults to randomly spend 3-week periods consuming either two whole-grain or refined grain rolls daily, there was no difference between the two treatments in terms of body weight, percentage of body fat, waist, or hip circumference [76].

Melanson et al compared the weight loss results of three groups:

1. Exercise only
2. Low-calorie diet containing whole-grains + exercise
3. Low-calorie diet containing no grains + exercise

After 12 weeks, the exercise-only group lost 1.64kg. The whole-grain group lost 4.7kg, and the no-grains group lost 5.0kg. At 24 weeks, the losses were 1.75, 5.7, and 6.2kg, respectively [77]. The differences between the whole-grain and no-cereal groups were not statistically significant.

Remember the WGC's dodgey citation of the whole-grain versus Slimfast study I mentioned some 5,780 words ago? Well, what the WGC kinda sorta for some strange reason forgot to mention, is that same study also compared the weight loss effects of the two starkly contrasting diets. Body weight fell by 3.2kg during the Slimfast diet, compared with 2.5kg during the whole-grain diet. Again, this difference was not statistically significant [78].

That leaves us with the recent study by Kristensen et al, which compared the effect of replacing refined wheat with whole-grain wheat for 12 weeks on body weight. The refined wheat group lost 2.7kg, compared to 3.6kg in the whole wheat group, a difference that once again was not statistically significant. Waist circumference decreased by 4.1cm in both groups. The only statistically significant difference the researchers could muster between the two groups was in the percentage of total fat loss. How big was this difference? Well, are you guys ready for it? I mean, it's pretty bloody huge, and I'm not sure you guys can handle such a mind-blowingly large figure!

You reckon you can, huh? Okay, tough guys (and girls), here it is...

Drum roll, please...

A massive, humungous, ginormous 0.9 percent more fat was lost in the whole-grain group! [79]

Yep, as a fat loss strategy, whole-grains are a complete waste of time. They're no better than refined grains, no grains, or Slimfast.

The Real Nitty Gritty-- Longer Term Trials

This is where we really grab whole-grains by the short and curlies and make those shifty little anti-nutrient-rich bastards squirm and squeal. This, ladies and gentlemen, is where we see if whole-grains, or the highly-touted cereal fibre they contain, truly do show any ability to lower actual disease or death rates.

Protection from cancer is a claim frequently made for high-fibre cereal foods; colon cancer in particular, we are repeatedly told, would be dramatically reduced if only we would all eat more whole-grains. Human poo contains toxins, and fibre speeds up the passage of this toxin-laden poo through our colorectal Route 66, thereby lowering our risk of cancer, so the story goes.

While confounder-prone epidemiological studies backing this notion are easy to find, none of the numerous randomized controlled intervention trials conducted in this area support the possibility that high cereal fibre intakes prevent the progression of colon cancer [80].

In fact, some of these trials noted worse outcomes in the treatment groups. In the four-year Polyp Prevention Trial, colorectal cancer was diagnosed in ten subjects from the high fibre group, and only four from the low-fibre group. Even after excluding those diagnosed within the first year of the study, the results were similarly unfavourable; four cases in the intervention group as compared to two in the control group. Polyp recurrence was virtually identical between the two groups [81].

In the three-year double-blind Phoenix Colon Cancer Prevention trial, there was a significantly higher proportion of subjects with three or more recurring polyps in the high-fibre group. Seven cases of colon cancer were reported in the high-fibre group, but only two in the low-fibre group. Those who have abandoned whole-grains and relished the subsequent improvements in gastrointestinal function would not be at all surprised to learn that the incidence of abdominal pain, intestinal gas, and abdominal bloating was significantly higher among those receiving the high-wheat fibre diet (as were nausea, diarrhoea and constipation) [82].

What About Cardiovascular Disease?

Well, the only study looking at the effect of increased cereal fibre on CVD incidence and mortality was the DART trial in the UK. That study, published in 1989, found that men randomized to eat more cereal fibre experienced a 27% relative risk increase in overall mortality and a 23% increase in the relative risk of CHD events at two years. These results did not reach statistical significance, but needless to say they hardly support the exuberant claims of the whole-grain crowd. The DART trial, the only one to put the "grain fibre = heart healthy" to the test, found it was a complete flop in preventing CHD or overall mortality [83].

And that's it. Over 40 years of sustained and relentless whole-grain propaganda, and the small handful of RCTs that lasted more than a few months show absolutely no disease or mortality benefit, and in fact suggest that over the longer term, cereal fibre will increase the risk of cancer, CHD, and overall mortality. That's a stark contrast to the results of the abundant episloppyology, so the whole-grain shills ignore the long-term RCTs along with the abundance of short-term RCTs that refute their beliefs, and instead focus on the confounder-prone rot that tells them what they want to hear. If the only people they deluded were themselves, this wouldn't be so bad. Unfortunately, millions of people around the world have fallen for the whole-grain scam, only to be met with either no improvement or a worsening of their health.

Don't you be one of them. You now know that the whole-grain thesis is a farce that benefits no one except cereal producers and the researchers they fund.

Hopefully, you've also learned something else important from this 2-part instalment, namely, the dangerously misleading nature of nutritional epidemiology. Statistics do not equal science, and associations do not equal cause-and-effect relationships.

You Call That a Benefit?

Before I go, there's something else I want to mention. This dissection has shown there is nothing to be gained from eating whole-grains, but it is true you may get a little something extra from brown rice. Unfortunately, that something extra happens to be a Group 1 carcinogen. You see, vitamins, minerals, amino acids and trace elements are not the only things plants absorb from the soil and water in which they grow. Toxic metals like arsenic also find their way into plants; analyses of hundreds of varieties of white and brown rice have found the latter to contain higher levels of arsenic than the former [84,85]. The higher concentration of arsenic in brown rice is attributed to the fact it still retains its outer layers; rice bran is an especially rich source of arsenic [86].

Numerous analyses of the arsenic content of rice have been published, and the results consistently show that Californian varieties contain lower levels of arsenic than rice grown in the southern US states of Arkansas, Louisiana, Mississippi, and Texas. Previous arsenic-based pesticide use on cotton fields now being used for rice production is believed to be the culprit [87]. Internationally, rice from Europe (Italy, Spain, France) also shows comparatively high arsenic levels [88,89].

What, if any, effect this has on human health is still a relatively understudied area, but I'd personally prefer to err on the side of caution. Along with avoiding brown rice, I also avoid rice from high-arsenic sources, and to further reduce arsenic content I use a high water:rice volume when cooking. A 2009 study found that a 6:1 water:rice ratio (i.e. using 6 cups of water to 1 cup of rice) removed 45% of arsenic in long-grain rice. The rice was boiled to eating texture and the remaining water discarded. Steaming was less consistent in reducing arsenic content, while low volume water cooking (2.5:1 water:rice ratio, boiled to dryness) failed to remove arsenic. Rinsing the rice prior to cooking produced a fourteen percent reduction in arsenic content, but the effect was only observed in basmati rice. The rinsing method employed was to place 100 grams of rice in 600 millilitres of distilled and deionised water and agitate the mixture routinely for three minutes. The water was then drained and the process repeated once more with a fresh batch of water [90]. An Indian study using similar water:rice ratios during cooking found similar results, but that a more extensive washing procedure (rinsing the rice 5-6 times until the discarded water became clear) removed 28% of arsenic [91].

But Anthony, I Need More Fibre!

I need to clear up something else before I sign off. This book is not anti-fibre, and neither am I. There are benefits to consuming a sensible level of dietary fibre, you know.

By increasing faecal bulk, for example, fibre promotes regularity and helps to prevent restroom visits degenerating into painful, vein-popping, teeth-clenching affairs that pit one's mental and physical fortitude against one's non-responsive bowels. That's pretty handy, especially if you'd rather die of old age in your sleep than prematurely haemorrhaging on the toilet.

Now, if you need to increase your fibre intake to reduce the risk of such an inglorious passing, I think the evidence clearly shows switching to whole-grains isn't the way to do it. Nope, just get your fibre from the same place humans got it from for the 2.4 million years or so before they started eating cereal grains.

Where would that be, you ask?

That would be fruits and vegetables, my little grasshoppers.

Yep, fibre can be found in abundance in fruits and vegetables, predominantly in soluble form as opposed to the mainly insoluble fibre found in cereal grains. Soluble fibre is more than capable of maintaining regular bowel function in humans, and has been efficiently doing so for millions of years. Soluble fibre is also more than capable of imparting satiating effects that curb appetite [92], with the additional benefit that fruits and especially vegetables tend to contain fewer calories than cereal grains.

There are other benefits to eating more fruits and veggies. Compare the pathetic inability of whole grains to improve antioxidant status with that of nutritionally superior fruit and vegetables. When young and older adult subjects doubled their usual intake of fruits and vegetables from 5 to 10 servings daily, substantial increases in blood antioxidant capacity were seen after 15 days [93]. In a Danish study, healthy males and females who consumed an extra 600 grams of fruit and vegetables daily for 25 days experienced reductions in lipoprotein oxidation and increases in the activity of glutathione peroxidase, an enzyme in the body that is a powerful scavenger of free radicals [94].

Vegetables, by the way, are the real Asian and Mediterranean secret to turning refined cereal grains into health foods. A couple of slices of white bread covered by jam or Hundreds n' Thousands is about as 'healthy' as a plate of freshly thawed cardboard. But get rid of the sugar-rich spreads and instead lace that bread with phenol-rich extra virgin olive oil, and smother it with a lightly fried mix of vegetables that includes onion, garlic, mushrooms, broccoli, and tomato--as the Greeks and Italians have been doing for eons--and you suddenly have an antioxidant, fibre- and nutrient-rich treat that is not only much healthier but also far tastier than any sawdust-like whole-grain. Ditto for Asian stir-fries. Keep the tasteless 'macrobiotic' brown rice... I'd rather eat a tasty, traditional white rice and veggie-rich Asian stir-fry any day, my friends.

Anyway, I'm Anthony Colpo and that was my short(ish) lesson for you on the whole-grain myth. I really hope you enjoyed it. Maybe not in a *"damn, this is better than sex and ice cream!"* kind of way, but more of a *"hey, I learned something pretty cool today!"* kinda way. Because it's very important to have both kinds of enjoyment in your lives, folks.

Ciao,

Anthony.

PS. One last, last thing: To say that bodybuilders like oats would be an understatement... they worship them.

I've never quite understood this religious-like reverence for oats... I mean, when people put oats in their protein shakes, things truly are getting a little bizarre. So what to do if you have been convinced by my whole-grain book but also belong to the Latter Day Church of Oat Worship? Easy. Pour out the required amount of oats into a bowl the night before you intend to eat them, cover them with water, then let them soak overnight. This will help neutralize many of the anti-nutrients; subsequent cooking will then really help kick those little mineral-binding, gut permeating bastards when they're down!

For obvious reasons, don't try this with whole-grain bread.

References

1. Story JA, Kritchevsky D. Denis Parsons Burkitt (1911-1993). *Journal of Nutrition*, 1994; 124: 1551-1554.
2. Rennie KL, et al. Estimating under-reporting of energy intake in dietary surveys using an individualised method. *British Journal of Nutrition*, 2007; 97: 1169–1176.
3. Goris AHC, et al. Undereating and underrecording of habitual food intake in obese men: selective underreporting of fat intake. *American Journal of Clinical Nutrition*, 2000; 71: 130–134.
4. Livingstone MB, et al. Accuracy of weighed dietary records in studies of diet and health. *British Medical Journal*, Mar 17, 1990; 300 (6726): 708-712.
5. Zacharski LR, et al. Decreased cancer risk after iron reduction in patients with peripheral arterial disease: results from a randomized trial. *Journal of the National Cancer Institute*, Jul 16, 2008; 100 (14): 996-1002.
6. Painter NS, Burkitt DP. Diverticular disease of the colon: a deficiency disease of western civilisation. *British Medical Journal*, May 22, 1971; 2: 450-454.
7. Burkitt DP. Dietary Fiber and Cancer. *Journal of Nutrition*, 1988; 118: 531-533.
8. Segal I, Walker AR. Low- fat intake with falling fibre intake commensurate with rarity of noninfective bowel disease in blacks in Soweto, Johannesburg, South Africa. *Nutrition and Cancer*, 1986; 8 (3): 185-191.
9. Hawk A. The Great Disease Enemy, Kak'ke (Beriberi) and the Imperial Japanese Army. *Military Medicine*, Apr 2006; 171 (4): 333-339.
10. Martel J, Raskin JB. History, incidence, and epidemiology of diverticulosis. *Journal of Clinical Gastroenterology*, 2008; 42: 1125-1127.

11. See: http://www.worldlifeexpectancy.com/country-health-profile/uganda (online access available as of Jan 2, 2014).

12. Painter NS. Diverticular disease of the colon. The first of the Western diseases shown to be due to a deficiency of dietary fibre. *South African Medical Journal*, Jun 26, 1982; 61 (26): 1016-1020.

13. Dodds C, et al. Effects of dietary fibre. *British Medical Journal*, Aug 19, 1972; 3 (5824): 472-473.

14. Painter NS, et al. Unprocessed bran in treatment of diverticular disease of the colon. *British Medical Journal*, 1972; 2: 137-140.

15. Brodribb AJ, Humphreys DM. Diverticular disease: three studies. Part II – Treatment with bran. *British Medical Journal*, 1976; 1: 425-428.

16. Brodribb AJ, Humphreys DM. Diverticular disease: three studies. Part III – Metabolic effect of bran in patients with diverticular disease. *British Medical Journal*, 1976; 1: 428-430.

17. Hyland JM, Taylor I. Does a high fibre diet prevent the complications of diverticular disease? *British Journal of Surgery*, 1980; 67: 77-79.

18. Leahy AL, et al. High fibre diet in symptomatic diverticular disease of the colon. *Annals of the Royal College of Surgeons of England*, 1985; 67: 173-174.

19. Brodribb AJ. Treatment of symptomatic diverticular disease with a high-fibre diet. *Lancet*, 1977; 1: 664-666.

20. Devroede G, et al. Medical management of diverticular disease: a random trial. *Gastroenterology*, 1977; 72: A134.

21. Hodgson WJH. The placebo effect. Is it important in diverticular disease? *American Journal of Gastroenterology*, 1977; 67: 157–162.

22. Ornstein MH et al. Are fibre supplements really necessary in diverticular disease of the colon? A controlled clinical trial. *British Medical Journal (Clinical Research Edition)*, 1981; 282 (6273): 1353-1356.

23. Ünlü C, et al. A systematic review of high-fibre dietary therapy in diverticular disease. *International Journal of Colorectal Disease*, 2012: 27: 419–427.
24. Seow CS, Seow-Choen F. High-fibre Diet and Colonic Diverticulosis. *Journal of Gastroenterology and Hepatology Research*, May 21, 2013; 2 (5): 561-563.
25. Biljkerk CJ, et al. Systematic review: the role of different types of fibre in the treatment of irritable bowel syndrome. *Alimentary Pharmacology & Therapeutics*, 2004; 19: 245–251.
26. Soltoft J, et al. A double-blind trial of the effect of wheat bran on symptoms of irritable bowel syndrome. *Lancet*, 1976; 307 (7954): 270-272. (Originally published as Volume 1, Issue 7954).
27. Peery AF, et al. A High-Fiber Diet Does Not Protect Against Asymptomatic Diverticulosis. *Gastroenterology*, Feb, 2012; 142 (2): 266-272.e1.
28. Aldoori WH. The protective role of dietary fiber in diverticular disease. *Advances in Experimental Medicine and Biology*, 1997; 427: 291-308.
29. Raina K, et al. Inositol hexaphosphate inhibits tumor growth, vascularity, and metabolism in TRAMP mice: a multiparametric magnetic resonance study. *Cancer Prevention Research*, Jan, 2013; 6 (1): 40-50.
30. Williams KA, et al. Protective effect of inositol hexaphosphate against UVB damage in HaCaT cells and skin carcinogenesis in SKH1 hairless mice. *Comparative Medicine*, Feb, 2011; 61 (1): 39-44.
31. Bacić I, et al. Efficacy of IP6 + inositol in the treatment of breast cancer patients receiving chemotherapy: prospective, randomized, pilot clinical study. *Journal of Experimental & Clinical Cancer Research*, Feb 12, 2010; 29: 12.
32. Kolappaswamy K, et al. Effect of inositol hexaphosphate on the development of UVB-induced skin tumors in SKH1 hairless mice. *Comparative Medicine*, Apr, 2009; 59 (2): 147-152.

33. Raina K, et al. Chemopreventive efficacy of inositol hexaphosphate against prostate tumor growth and progression in TRAMP mice. *Clinical Cancer Research*, May 15, 2008; 14 (10): 3177-3184.

34. Vucenik I, et al. Comparison of pure inositol hexaphosphate and high-bran diet in the prevention of DMBA-induced rat mammary carcinogenesis. *Nutrition and Cancer*, 1997; 28 (1): 7-13.

35. Jacobs DR Jr, et al. Whole-grain intake may reduce the risk of ischemic heart disease death in postmenopausal women: the Iowa Women's Health Study. *American Journal of Clinical Nutrition*, 1998; 68: 248–257.

36. Herms DA, WJ Mattson. The dilemma of plants: to grow or to defend. *Quarterly Review of Biology*, 1992; 67: 283-335.

37. Coley PD, et al. Resource availability and antiherbivore defense. *Science*, Nov 22, 1985; 230 (4728): 895-899.

38. Freed DLJ. Lectins in food: their importance in health and disease. *Journal of Nutritional Medicine*, 1991; 2: 45-64.

39. Brady PG, et al. Identification of the dietary lectin, wheat germ agglutinin, in human intestinal contents. *Gastroenterology*, Aug, 1978; 75 (2): 236-239.

40. Wang Q, et al. Identification of intact peanut lectin in peripheral venous blood. *Lancet*, 1998; 352 (9143): 1831-1832.

41. Pusztai A, et al. Antinutritive effects of wheat-germ agglutinin and other N-acetylglucosamine-specific lectins. *British Journal of Nutrition*, Jul, 1993; 70 (1): 313-321.

42. Ryder SD, et al. Peanut ingestion increases rectal proliferation in individuals. *Gastroenterology*, 1998; 114: 44-49.

43. Bohn T, et al. Phytic acid added to white-wheat bread inhibits fractional apparent magnesium absorption in humans. American Journal of Clinical Nutrition, Mar, 2004; (79) 3: 418-423.

44. Torre M, et al. Effects of dietary fiber and phytic acid on mineral availability. *Critical Reviews in Food Science and Nutrition*, 1991; 30 (1): 1-22.
45. Reinhold JG, et al. Effects of purified phytate and phytate-rich bread upon metabolism of zinc, calcium, phosphorous, and nitrogen in man. *Lancet*, Feb 10, 1973; 1 (7798): 283-288.
46. Ervin RB, et al. Dietary intakes of selected minerals for the United States population: 1999-2000. *Advance Data*, Apr 27, 2004; 341: 1-5.
47. Ford ES, Mokdad, AH. Dietary Magnesium Intake in a National Sample of U.S. Adults. *Journal of Nutrition*, 2003; 133: 2879-2882.
48. Hambidge M. Human zinc deficiency. *Journal of Nutrition*, May, 2000; 130 (Suppl. 5): 1344S-1349S.
49. GM Berlyne, et al. Bedouin osteomalacia due to calcium deprivation caused by high phytic acid content of unleavened bread. *American Journal of Clinical Nutrition*, Sep 1973; 26: 910 – 911.
50. Zoppi G, et al. Potential complications in the use of wheat bran for constipation in infancy. *Journal of Pediatric Gastroenterology and Nutrition*, 1982; 1 (1): 91-95.
51. Sandstead HH. Fiber, phytates and mineral nutrition. *Nutrition Reviews*, 1992; 50: 30-31.
52. Reynolds RD. Bioavailability of vitamin B6 from plant foods. *American Journal of Clinical Nutrition*, 1988; 48: 863-867.
53. Kabir H, et al. Comparative vitamin B-6 bioavailability from tuna, whole wheat bread and peanut butter. *Journal of Nutrition*, 1983; 113: 2412-2420.
54. Gregory JF. Bioavailability of vitamin B6 in nonfat dry milk and a fortified rice breakfast cereal product. *Journal of Food Science*, 1980; 45: 84-86.
55. Leklem JE, et al. Bioavailability of vitamin B6 from wheat bread in humans. *Journal of Nutrition*, 1980; 110: 1819-1828.

56. Lindberg AS, et al. The effect of wheat bran on the bioavailability of vitamin B6 in young men. *Journal of Nutrition*, 1983; 113: 2578-2586.
57. Ewer TK. Rachitogenicity of green oats. *Nature*, 1950; 166: 732-733.
58. Hidiroglou M, et al. Effect of a single intramuscular dose of vitamin D on concentrations of liposoluble vitamins in the plasma of heifers winter-fed oat silage, grass silage or hay. *Canadian Journal of Animal Science*, 1980; 60: 311-318.
59. Batchelor AJ, Compston JE: Reduced plasma half-life of radio-labelled 25-hydroxyvitamin D3 in subjects receiving a high fiber diet. *British Journal of Nutrition*, 1983; 49 (2): 213-216.
60. Cullumbine H, et al. Mineral Metabolism on Rice Diets. *British Journal of Nutrition*, 1950; 4: 101-111.
61. Rama Rao G, et al. The effect of the degree of polishing of rice on nitrogen and mineral metabolism in human subjects. *Cereal Chemistry*, Jan-Feb, 1960; 37 (1): 71-78.
62. Reinhold JG, et al. Decreased Absorption of Calcium, Magnesium, Zinc and Phosphorus by Humans due to Increased Fiber and Phosphorus Consumption as Wheat Bread. *Journal of Nutrition*, 1976; 106: 493-503.
63. Miyoshi H, et al. Effects of brown rice on apparent digestibility and balance of nutrients in young men on low protein diets. *Journal of Nutritional Science and Vitaminology*, 1987; 33: 207-218.
64. Williams VR, et al. Rice Starch, Varietal Differences in Amylose Content of Rice Starch. *Journal of Agricultural and Food Chemistry*, 1958; 6 (1): 47–48.
65. Miller JB, et al. Rice: a high or low glycemic food? *American Journal of Clinical Nutrition*, 1992; 56: 1034-1036.
66. Zhang G, et al. Substituting white rice with brown rice for 16 weeks does not substantially affect metabolic risk factors in middle-aged Chinese men and women with diabetes or a high risk for diabetes. *Journal of Nutrition*, Sep, 2011; 141 (9): 1685-1690.

67. Jenkins DJA, et al. Wholemeal versus wholegrain breads: proportion of whole or cracked grain and the glycaemic response. *British Medical Journal*, Oct 15, 1988; 297: 958-960.

68. Heaton KW, et al. Particle size of wheat, maize, and oat test meals: effects on plasma glucose and insulin responses and on the rate of starch digestion in vitro. *American Journal of Clinical Nutrition*, 1988; 47: 675-682.

69. Najjar AM, et al. The acute impact of ingestion of breads of varying composition on blood glucose, insulin and incretins following first and second meals. *British Journal of Nutrition*, 2009; 101: 391–398.

70. Giacco R, et al. Effects of rye and whole wheat versus refined cereal foods on metabolic risk factors: A randomised controlled two-centre intervention study. *Clinical Nutrition*, Dec, 2013; 32 (6): 941-949.

71. Andersson A, et al. Whole-Grain Foods Do Not Affect Insulin Sensitivity or Markers of Lipid Peroxidation and Inflammation in Healthy, Moderately Overweight Subjects. *Journal of Nutrition*, 2007; 137: 1401–1407.

72. Jenkins DJ, et al. Effect of wheat bran on glycemic control and risk factors for cardiovascular disease in type 2 diabetes. *Diabetes Care*, Sep, 2002; 25 (9): 1522-1528.

73. Enright L, Slavin J. No effect of 14 day consumption of whole grain diet compared to refined grain diet on antioxidant measures in healthy, young subjects: a pilot study. *Nutrition Journal*, Mar 19, 2010; 9: 12.

74. Brownlee IA, et al. Markers of cardiovascular risk are not changed by increased whole-grain intake: the WHOLEheart study, a randomised, controlled dietary intervention. *British Journal of Nutrition*, 2010; 104: 125–134.

75. Katcher HI, et al. The effects of a whole grain–enriched hypocaloric diet on cardiovascular disease risk factors in men and women with metabolic syndrome. *American Journal of Clinical Nutrition*, 2008; 87: 79–90.

76. Bodinham CL, et al. Short-term effects of whole-grain wheat on appetite and food intake in healthy adults: a pilot study. *British Journal of Nutrition*, 2011; 106: 327–330.

77. Melanson KJ, et al. Consumption of Whole-Grain Cereals during Weight Loss: Effects on Dietary Quality, Dietary Fiber, Magnesium, Vitamin B-6, and Obesity. *Journal of the American Dietetic Association*, 2006; 106: 1380-1388.

78. Rave K, et al. Improvement of insulin resistance after diet with a whole-grain based dietary product: results of a randomized, controlled cross-over study in obese subjects with elevated fasting blood glucose. *British Journal of Nutrition*, 2007; 98: 929–936.

79. Kristensen M, et al. Whole Grain Compared with Refined Wheat Decreases the Percentage of Body Fat Following a 12-Week, Energy-Restricted Dietary Intervention in Postmenopausal Women. *Journal of Nutrition*, 2012; 142: 710–716.

80. Asano T, McLeod RS. Dietary fibre for the prevention of colorectal adenomas and carcinomas (Cochrane Review). In: *The Cochrane Library*, Issue 2, 2002. Oxford.

81. Schatzkin A, et al. Lack of effect of a low-fat, high-fiber diet on the recurrence of colorectal adenomas. *New England Journal of Medicine*, Apr 20, 2000; 342 (16): 1149-1155.

82. Alberts DS, et al. Lack of effect of a high fiber cereal supplement on the recurrence of colorectal adenomas. *New England Journal of Medicine*, Apr 20, 2000; 342 (16): 1156-1162.

83. Burr ML, et al. Effects of changes in fat, fish, and fibre intakes on death and myocardial reinfarction: diet and reinfarction trial (DART). *Lancet*, 1989; 2: 757-761.

84. Meharg AA, et al. Speciation and localization of arsenic in white and brown rice grains. *Environmental Science & Technology*, Feb 15, 2008; 42(4): 1051-1057.

85. Zavala YJ, Duxbury JM. Arsenic in rice: I. Estimating normal levels of total arsenic in rice grain. *Environmental Science & Technology*, May 15, 2008; 42 (10): 3856-3860.

86. Sun GX, et al. Inorganic Arsenic in Rice Bran and Its Products Are an Order of Magnitude Higher than in Bulk Grain. *Environmental Science & Technology*, 2008; 42 (19): 7542–7546.

87. Williams PN, et al. Market Basket Survey Shows Elevated Levels of As in South Central U.S. Processed Rice Compared to California: Consequences for Human Dietary Exposure. *Environmental Science & Technology*, 2007; 41: 2178-2183.

88. Zavala YJ, Duxbury JM. Arsenic in rice: I. Estimating normal levels of total arsenic in rice grain. *Environmental Science & Technology*, May 15, 2008; 42 (10): 3856-3860.

89. Meharg AA, et al. Geographical variation in total and inorganic arsenic content of polished (white) rice. *Environmental Science & Technology*, Mar 1, 2009; 43 (5): 1612-1617.

90. Raab A, et al. Cooking rice in a high water to rice ratio reduces inorganic arsenic content. *Journal of Environmental Monitoring*, 2009; 11: 41-44.

91. Sengupta MK, et al. Arsenic burden of cooked rice: traditional and modern methods. *Food Chemical Toxicology*, 2006; 44: 1823-1829.

92. Howarth NC, et al. Dietary fiber and weight regulation. *Nutrition Reviews*, May 2001; 59 (5): 129-139.

93. Cao G, et al. Increases in human plasma antioxidant capacity after consumption of controlled diets high in fruit and vegetables. *American Journal of Clinical Nutrition*, 1998; 68: 1081-1087.

94. Dragsted LO, et al. The 6-a-day study: effects of fruit and vegetables on markers of oxidative stress and antioxidative defense in healthy nonsmokers. *American Journal of Clinical Nutrition*, 2004; 79: 1060-1072.

Free Excerpt from *The Fat Loss Bible*

Are Protein and Animal Fats Dangerous?

Claim 1: Animal Fats Cause Heart Disease.

I could write an entire book debunking the claim that animal fats cause heart disease. In fact, I already have. My book *The Great Cholesterol Con* absolutely destroys every possible defence of the ludicrous cholesterol/saturated fat theory of heart disease. This theory claims that saturated fatty acids from animal and tropical fats cause heart disease both directly and indirectly via cholesterol elevation. This theory portrays cholesterol as a deadly artery-clogging toxin, when in fact it is an essential component of our cells that we simply could not live without. Did you know that your brain and nervous system are especially rich in cholesterol? How on Earth did humans survive for 2.4 million years if two of the most essential components of their physiology were comprised of such a deadly substance?

I'll now outline a greatly condensed explanation of why the anti-cholesterol, anti-animal fat campaign is a complete fraud. If you want a far more thorough and fully referenced destruction of this spurious campaign, you can consult *The Great Cholesterol Con*.

The modern anti-cholesterol mania was ignited primarily by a single disgruntled researcher by the name of Ancel Keys, who in the early 1950s used atrociously one-sided data in order to support his preconceived theory that fat caused heart disease. Keys placed six countries on a graph and was able to display a strong positive linear association between their fat intake and per capita CHD rates. In other words, as fat intake went up so too did CHD mortality.

But his comparison was a complete sham; data for twenty-two countries were actually available at the time, and when all these countries were considered the relationship between fat intake and CHD disappeared. Furthermore, it was possible to selectively pull six alternate countries from the list and show a negative association in which increasing fat intake was associated with *reduced* CHD mortality!

Researchers who pointed all this out were simply ignored, and Keys subsequently received funding to perform a large epidemiological study known as the Seven Countries Study. Once more, the countries were hand-picked by Keys and showed that total fat as well as cholesterol levels were associated with CHD mortality. But what was ignored was that *within* these countries the associations disappeared. Intra-country comparisons are more relevant than cross-country comparisons, as the residents share far more similar political, cultural and dietary habits – all of which can have a profound impact on health and longevity. But again, Keys' flawed conclusions were taken at face value and allowed to steer the entire field of coronary disease prevention down the wrong path, with disastrous consequences.

We are repeatedly told saturated fat has been proven to cause heart disease. This claim is absurd. Again, why would nature see fit to include such a toxic substance in our ancestral diet, and how did our species survive for millions of years if it was so deadly? In *The Great Cholesterol Con,* I list all the epidemiological studies that have followed population groups for extended periods of time and tracked their saturated fat intake. Over two dozen such studies have been published, but only 4 have even been able to detect desperately weak associations between saturated fat intake and increased heart disease mortality. Another of these studies found increased saturated fat intake associated with reduced heart disease mortality, whilst the remaining twenty-one studies found no association whatsoever.

Most importantly of all, numerous dietary intervention trials have been conducted in which subjects were randomly assigned to follow low saturated fat diets or diets higher in saturated fat. These trials have completely failed to show any benefit whatsoever for saturated fat restriction or dietary cholesterol lowering on heart disease incidence or mortality. In some of those studies, the subjects eating the so-called 'healthy' cholesterol-lowering diets actually suffered higher rates of heart disease and/or cancer!

We are repeatedly told that science has established a rock-solid link between high cholesterol and CHD, but autopsy studies have repeatedly failed to show any relationship between blood cholesterol levels and the degree of atherosclerosis in the deceased arteries. Individuals with very low cholesterol levels have been found to have arteries riddled with atherosclerosis, and vice versa.

In the face of such dismal scientific support, it's no wonder that cholesterol-lowering statin drugs have been warmly embraced by the medical establishment. After all, they are very effective for lowering cholesterol and have reduced CHD incidence in numerous trials. But as I explain in *The Great Cholesterol Con* and a 2005 *Journal of American Physicians and Surgeons* paper (freely available online at http://www.jpands.org/vol10no3/colpo.pdf), statin drugs produce this effect not by cholesterol reduction but by mechanisms unrelated to lipid lowering[1].

I cannot emphasize enough that the anti-animal fat, anti-cholesterol campaign is a complete farce, one that deserves to die the quickest and most decisive possible death. Its devastating consequences go far beyond simply scaring people away from perfectly healthy eggs and succulent cuts of meat. The real tragedy is that the real causes of CHD are largely ignored by most researchers and medical practitioners and therefore result in millions of unnecessary deaths each year (in 2008 alone, an estimated an estimated 7.3 million deaths worldwide were due to CHD)[2].

Iron-Clad Evidence that Cholesterol is Not the Problem

Much ado is made about the low CHD rates of the French, the Japanese, the Inuit Eskimo, etcetera, but premenopausal women all around the world enjoy very low rates of heart disease - even those living in

Western countries where CHD is the number one killer. In fact, in modernized nations pre-menopausal women enjoy the lowest mortality rates of any adult group. But when women reach menopause, the honeymoon suddenly ends and their risk of cardiovascular disease rises sharply to match that of men the same age.

For years this phenomenon was attributed to the primary female reproductive hormone estrogen, which allegedly exerted some sort of protective effect that scientists could never actually pinpoint or satisfactorily explain.

The estrogen theory was wrong, and discredited by published research as far back as 1978. In the famous Framingham study, researchers observed that when a pre-menopausal woman underwent hysterectomy removing the uterus only - the component of her reproductive organs that sheds its lining and loses blood each month – but left her estrogen-producing ovaries intact, her risk of heart disease rose just as sharply as when both her uterus *and* ovaries were removed[3].

So if her estrogen levels remained intact but her heart disease risk still jumped skyward, then this increased risk must somehow be related to the fact that her menstrual cycle stopped permanently. Before I reveal the relationship, I'll quickly mention one other important piece of evidence that blows the estrogen hypothesis out of the water: In 2002, the results of two large-scale clinical trials using estrogen and progestin were published. One of these showed no reduction in either primary or secondary CHD events in women taking the two hormones, while another was stopped early after researchers observed an *increase* in CHD, stroke and breast cancer in the HRT group[4,5]. In 2004, the published results of a trial using estrogen only also failed to show any protection against CHD[6].

So much for the estrogen theory. And it certainly isn't low cholesterol levels that are protecting premenopausal women; study after study has found CHD has little relationship with cholesterol in women. One of the more recent examples is the 10-year HUNT 2 study in Norway that included 27,852 women aged 20–74 years. It found that, as cholesterol went up, the risk of cardiovascular disease (CHD, heart failure and stroke) declined. When coronary heart disease mortality was examined in isolation, the association with cholesterol appeared to follow a U-shaped curve. The lowest CHD risk was seen between 5.0-6.9 mmol/l (193-267 mg/dl), which hardly supports the simple-minded "lower is better" mentality that has come to dominate the CHD prevention arena. And most importantly, those with a reading over 7.0 mmol/l (270 mg/dl) enjoyed a 28 percent relative risk reduction in overall mortality compared with women whose cholesterol was under 5.0 mmol/l. This risk was determined after adjusting for age, smoking and systolic blood pressure[7].

Currently, the most accurate and widely used indicator of bodily iron status is *serum ferritin*, which measures the concentration of iron in the blood. In teenage males and females, serum ferritin levels average around 21-23 mcg/l. This rises to around 94 mcg/l in males aged 18-45, and 124 mcg/l in men over 45, but remains in the vicinity of 25 mcg/l among premenopausal women. After menopause, where menstruation comes to a permanent halt and the female CHD risk rises to match that seen in age-matched males, the average serum ferritin level is around 89 mcg/l[8,9].

So far, two clinical trials have been conducted examining the effect of iron-lowering upon CHD incidence and mortality. The first of these was the FeAST trial, in which vascular disease patients were assigned to a placebo group or to have regular phlebotomy (blood withdrawal). The phlebotomy group reduced their average serum ferritin level from 125 mcg/l to 52 mcg/l, and only one person (3.4 percent) experienced an adverse cardiovascular event (angioplasty). In the control group, eight patients (42 percent) experienced heart attack, heart failure, unstable angina, or dysrhythmia[10].

The second was a larger and longer-running trial involving peripheral artery disease patients. The designated serum ferritin goal in the phlebotomy group was 25 mcg/l, but in reality was reduced from an average of 122 mcg/l to only 80 mcg/l. As a result of this lacklustre attempt at iron reduction, there was a 15 percent reduction in overall mortality and a 12 percent reduction in the composite endpoint of death and non-fatal heart attack/stroke that did not reach statistical significance. However, in the youngest age quartile (ages 43-61), there was an impressive 53 percent reduction in overall mortality and a 59 percent reduction in the composite endpoint of death and non-fatal heart attack and stroke. In this instance, the differences were indeed statistically significant[11].

A subsequent report from the same trial found that, in addition to lowered CHD risk, there was also a significantly lower incidence of cancer among those who received phlebotomy. Patients in the iron reduction group were 35 percent less likely to develop cancer. Among the study participants who did develop cancer, those in the iron reduction group had 61 percent lower cancer-specific and 51 percent lower all-cause mortality, respectively[12].

That such impressive results were noted even when the degree of iron reduction was woefully inadequate indicates that iron reduction has the potential to save millions of lives around the world. Iron reduction, when performed under medical guidance, is a low-cost therapy that produces little to no adverse effects. And it remains almost entirely ignored by the medical profession. This, dear readers, is the most devastating aspect of the travesty that constitutes the cholesterol hypothesis of heart disease. Those that continue to defend this theory are effectively defending a misleading smokescreen that results in millions of unnecessary deaths each year.

For those who wish to learn more about the pivotal role of supposedly 'normal' iron levels in chronic disease, I strongly recommend *Exposing the Hidden Dangers of Iron* by Drs. Weinberg and Garrison (Cumberland House Publishing). Written for medical professionals but easily accessed and understood by laypeople, this outstanding book answers almost every question you could possibly think of regarding iron and iron reduction.

False Claim 2: Animal Protein and Fat Cause Cancer

If meat caused cancer, then vegetarians should consistently display lower rates of cancer than their omnivorous counterparts.

They don't.

The studies most frequently cited in support of vegetarian diets have involved Seventh-day Adventists living in California. Scientific interest in this population was inspired by data from the early seventies showing that, as a group, Seventh-day Adventists enjoyed a significantly lower death rate from cancer than non-Adventists. Members of this religion are exhorted to abstain from alcohol and tobacco, and most also shun the use of pork products. In addition, approximately one-half of Seventh-Day Adventists follow a lacto-ovo vegetarian diet, using vegetables, fruits, whole grains and nuts abundantly while avoiding the use of tea and coffee.

A recent study of over 34,000 Californian Seventh-Day Adventists, published in 1999, found that vegetarians had lower risks of hypertension, diabetes, arthritis, colon cancer, prostate cancer, fatal CHD in males, and death from all causes. Again, vegetarians displayed a number of healthful dietary habits unrelated to meat intake that were not shared by their omnivorous brethren. Vegetarians consumed more tomatoes, nuts, and fruit, but less coffee and donuts than non-vegetarians. Non-vegetarian Seventh-Day Adventists also consumed alcoholic beverages twenty times more frequently than their vegetarian counterparts[13]. As an earlier study of Adventists published in 1975, these observations clearly showed that those who shunned meat also adopted other dietary measures that protected their health[14].

Reinforcing this notion was the fact that, along with many of the aforementioned disorders, obesity increased as meat consumption increased. Obesity is well known to confer an increased risk of heart disease and cancer. Meat consumption, however, has nothing whatsoever to do with the accumulation of excess body fat; as we saw in Chapter 18, study after study has repeatedly failed to find any weight or fat loss advantage for vegetarian diets. The greater meat consumption of obese Seventh-Day Adventists was simply one of numerous characteristics present with greater frequency among those living less healthy lifestyles. Why single out meat when so many other possible culprits were present?

When we take a look at other large-scale studies involving populations other than Seventh-Day Adventists that recruited vegetarians and non-vegetarians and compared their subsequent mortality rates, the picture changes dramatically.

Three such studies have been conducted, all from the UK: the Health Food Shoppers Study, the Oxford Vegetarian Study and the EPIC-Oxford Study. The Health Food Shoppers Study, involving almost 10,000 health food store patrons in England, found a similar all-cause death rate among vegetarians and omnivores after seventeen years[15].

The Oxford Vegetarian Study compared over 6,800 vegetarians and non-vegetarians and found a 20 percent reduction in overall mortality among the former after 12 years[16]. More recent follow-up by the Oxford authors, however, found that the reduction in overall mortality had disappeared. In fact, the only significant difference remaining for any cause of death was seen for mental and neurological diseases, which were 2.5 times higher among vegetarians[17].

A 2003 report on the EPIC-Oxford Study, involving 56,000 subjects, also found no difference in overall mortality between vegetarians and omnivores after 5.9 years. Vegetarians displayed slightly higher mortality from all cancers and stroke[18].

A more recent paper on the EPIC study, with follow-up to 2007 and this time encompassing over 64,000 participants, again found no difference in overall mortality between vegetarians and non-vegetarians. Fish eaters and vegetarians had slightly lower rates of coronary heart disease than meat eaters, but higher rates of stroke. Total cancer incidence was significantly lower among fish eaters and borderline significantly lower among vegetarians than among meat eaters. In stark contrast to prevailing anti-meat dogma, the risk of colorectal cancer was significantly higher among vegetarians. For all causes of death combined, mortality in fish eaters was non-significantly lower than in meat eaters, while mortality in vegetarians was non-significantly higher[19].

Contrary to popular claims, the above studies show vegetarianism offered no real protection from cancer and did not confer any mortality advantage. This is despite the fact that the vegetarians in the Health Food Shoppers and Oxford studies were less likely to be cigarette smokers. In the Oxford study, vegetarians weighed less, drank less alcohol and exercised more. Information about exercise habits was not available for EPIC-Oxford, but vegetarians in this study were less likely to be heavy smokers or overweight.

Another study commonly used in support of vegetarianism was conducted by the German Cancer Research Center. In 1978 researchers from the center began following 1,904 vegetarians, 225 of whom died over the next eleven years. Normally, 470 deaths would have been expected in a sample of typical Germans.

This study, however, could not even begin to be used by any rational commentator as evidence that meat avoidance is beneficial. For starters, when the researchers compared death rates among strict vegetarians who never ate meat and 'moderate' vegetarians who occasionally ate meat or fish, they found similar cancer, cardiovascular disease and all-cause mortality rates among the two groups.

Furthermore, only four percent of males and three percent of females in the study were smokers; the corresponding figures for the rest of Germany were 41 and 26 percent, respectively. The vegetarians in the study were generally better educated and were more likely to be employed in professional jobs than the general population. They were also far less likely to be overweight[20]. Little surprise, then, that this group experienced lower mortality than the general population!

When the authors examined the effect of various confounding factors, they found that the strongest predictor by far of reduced all-cause and cardiovascular mortality was a higher level of physical activity[21].

The German study merely adds to the considerable volume of evidence showing that being physically active, avoiding overweight and eschewing cigarettes all increase longevity. The claim that shunning a nutrient-packed food like meat contributes to an increase in life span, through some bizarre twist of biochemistry, is a shameless exercise in junk science.

It should also be pointed out that studies examining meat-eaters who follow healthier-than-usual lifestyles have revealed mortality rates similar to or superior to those seen in the aforementioned vegetarian studies. An 8-year follow-up of over 5,200 Californian Mormon high priests found 53 percent lower cancer mortality, a 48 percent reduction in cardiovascular deaths, and 53 percent lower all-cause mortality than the rest of the white California population. For middle-aged high priests adhering to the three important health practices of never smoking cigarettes, engaging in regular physical activity and getting proper sleep, the reductions were even more impressive; cancer, cardiovascular and total deaths were reduced by 66, 86 and 78 percent, respectively![22]

In another Californian study, this time involving residents of Alameda County, 10 years of follow-up revealed that the strongest predictors of survival were:

1) never smoking cigarettes; 2) regular physical activity; 3) moderate or no use of alcohol; 4) attaining seven to eight hours of sleep per day, and; 5) maintaining proper weight[23].

Despite the vociferous claims of vegetarian activists, who have shown themselves to be in no way averse to bending the truth when it suits their agenda, the fact remains that vegetarianism has not been demonstrated to offer any reduction in cancer or all-cause mortality - even when using the garbage-laden modern Western diet as the reference standard!

False Claim 3: High Protein Intakes Cause Kidney Damage

There is evidence that a high protein intake may be harmful to people with pre-existing kidney damage. Protein metabolism results in the production of urea, which must be filtered through the kidneys. Individuals suffering impaired function may not be able to safely process the increased amounts of urea on a high-protein diet.

But does this mean individuals with healthy kidneys should also avoid higher protein intakes?

A study with twenty bodybuilders and 18 other highly-trained individuals examined the effects of high-protein diets on kidney function. Some of the subjects in the study were consuming up to 2.8g/kg of protein daily (210g protein daily for a 75kg individual). Such intakes would have a lot of orthodox nutritionists in a fit, but all measures of kidney function fell within normal ranges[24].

A comparison of healthy subjects eating 100g or more of protein per day with long-term vegetarians eating 30g or less of protein per day concluded that both groups had similar kidney function. The subjects were aged 30-80 and both groups displayed similar progressive deterioration of kidney function with age[25].

Empirically, bodybuilders and strength athletes have been consuming high-protein diets for decades. Given the widespread global participation in these activities, if the claims of kidney damage were true, by now there would be an enormous number of case studies of ex-bodybuilders and strength athletes afflicted with kidney disease. Needless to say, this is not the case.

High-protein diets may even be of benefit to advanced kidney disease patients, so long as they meet certain important criteria. A clinical trial by Californian researchers compared a low-iron, moderate-carbohydrate but *ad libitum* protein (derived from white meats, eggs, and dairy) diet with the low-protein, high-carbohydrate diet traditionally used with kidney patients. The special diet was designed to reduce glycation and also produced a substantial reduction in iron stores (via avoidance of iron-rich red meats and consumption of foods containing iron-binding agents). The mean serum ferritin level in the treatment group plummeted from 301 mcg/l to 36 mcg/l. Over a period of almost four years, those on the special low-iron diet were 50 percent less likely to either die or deteriorate to point where they required dialysis[26]. This an extremely impressive result given that chronic kidney disease typically has a poor prognosis and that modern medicine has little to offer in the way of effective treatments.

False Claim 4: High Protein Intakes Weaken Bones and Cause Osteoporosis

Before we dismantle this myth, we need to quickly get up to speed on the concepts of *acid-base balance* and *metabolic acidosis*. Acid-base imbalance occurs when blood pH shifts out of the normal range (7.35 to 7.45); an excess of acid is called *acidosis* and an excess of base is called *alkalosis*. The body has inbuilt mechanisms to keep blood pH in a tight range, and when the pH balance tips too far towards the acidic end of the spectrum a phenomenon known as metabolic acidosis results.

Meats, along with cereal grains, are acid-forming foods. In controlled feeding experiments, diets high in animal or purified proteins have often caused increased calcium excretion. Some researchers have long held that this calcium (an alkaline mineral) was being shed from bone in an attempt by the body to counter increased acidity in the bloodstream. Over time this protein-induced 'leaching' of calcium from the skeletal system could lead to significant decreases in bone mineral density, increasing the risk of osteoporosis.

Well, that's the theory. In real life, however, it is low-protein intakes that are generally associated with poorer bone health. A recent review of the scientific research in this area, headed by researcher Jane E. Kerstetter from the University of Connecticut, found several lines of evidence strongly contradicting the high-protein-diets-cause-bone-loss theory:

Many epidemiological studies have found a significant positive relationship between protein intake and bone mass or density. The vast majority examined older adults and generally observed a positive association between dietary protein and bone health.

In studies examining the fate of radioactive calcium isotopes, greater calcium absorption is seen with higher dietary protein (from meat) when daily calcium intake is 600-800 milligrams. At higher calcium intakes, no positive (nor detrimental) effect of high-protein diets is observed.

Meta-analysis of randomized, placebo-controlled trials found an overall slightly positive impact of protein supplementation (from all different sources) on lumbar bone mineral density. These small changes, however, did not translate to a beneficial association between dietary protein and fracture rates; no significant association (either positive or negative) of protein intake with fracture incidence was found.

Meta-analysis of the relationship between dietary acid generating capacity and urinary calcium, calcium balance, and markers of bone resorption (break down of bone and subsequent mineral loss into the bloodstream) predictably observed a significant positive relationship between net acid excretion (NAE) and urinary calcium. But NAE was not associated with calcium balance nor markers of bone resorption.

A number of studies have found significantly greater levels of IGF-1 in participants consuming the higher protein diets. The anabolic effect of IGF-1 on muscle, which in turn could exert a beneficial effect on bone health, may help further explain the positive relationship between dietary protein and bone (changes in bone mass and muscle strength tend to correlate over one's lifespan).

Kerstetter and her colleagues concluded: *"The recommendation to intentionally restrict dietary protein to improve bone health is unwarranted, and potentially even dangerous to those individuals who consume inadequate protein."*[27].

More Vegan Nonsense

The most vocal proponents of the protein-causes-bone-loss theory are those who promote vegetarian and vegan diets. These commentators rail not just against protein, but specifically animal protein. Animal protein, they assure us, is a major cause of the high rates of osteoporosis seen in Western countries.

Once again, if their claims were correct, we would expect to see higher bone densities in vegetarian and vegan individuals. In fact, the opposite is true. Studies repeatedly show either no difference or *lower* bone densities in those who follow vegetarian diets.

A recent meta-analysis encompassing nine studies of 2749 subjects (1880 women and 869 men) found that, overall, bone mineral density was 4 percent lower in vegetarians than in omnivores at both the femoral neck and the lumbar spine. The effect was more pronounced in vegans, who totally avoid animal products. While the researchers concluded *"the effect size is unlikely to result in a clinically important increase in fracture risk"*, the results do not even begin to support the incessant and rather shrill claims by vegetarian/vegan activists that meat and animal protein are harmful to bones[28].

A 2006 review that focused solely on veganism found a statistically significant correlation between decreased animal protein ingestion and low bone density in the hip area. The consistency of this finding was especially noteworthy when considered in light of the varied geographic locations of the studies (Finland, Taiwan and the USA). When it came to animal protein intake and fracture risk, conflicting data were observed; some studies reported an inverse correlation, while others found a positive association. Body mass index showed a more consistent relationship, with lower BMI associated with increased fracture risk. Individuals whose strict vegan diets cause them to consume insufficient calories and maintain low body weights may well be at increased risk of fracture; muscle and fat place extra stress on the skeleton, forcing an adaptive strengthening response. Higher muscle mass may also contribute to greater co-ordination and decreased risk of falls[29].

Ketogenic Diets: Exception to the Rule?

Despite their physically active lifestyles, Alaskan Eskimos were shown to have lower bone density and an earlier and more intense onset of bone loss than citizens of modernized and far more sedentary USA[30]. The Eskimos follow a very high-protein diet low in fresh plant matter; whether it is their very low carbohydrate intake, low calcium intake, or scarcity of alkalinizing fresh plant foods that contributes to their earlier and faster bone loss is unclear.

Scientists from the University of Chicago examined the effect of a very-low-carbohydrate diet on acid-base balance, kidney-stone risk, and calcium and bone metabolism. The researchers hypothesized that in addition to the effects of a high-protein intake alone, a low-carbohydrate diet could provide an exaggerated acid load through incomplete oxidation of fat and resultant ketone production. Ten healthy subjects consumed their usual diet then followed the Atkins diet for 6 weeks. This included Atkins' prescribed two-week *"induction"* phase followed by a moderately carbohydrate-restricted maintenance diet for 4 weeks. Compared with the usual diet, the Atkins diet delivered nearly twofold greater protein and fat intakes. Amounts of calcium, magnesium, sodium, potassium, and chloride did not differ significantly among the diets. The induction and maintenance diets had significantly greater contents of phosphorus, sulphur, and acid ash compared with the usual diet.

As expected, urine acidity and calcium excretion markedly increased during the induction and maintenance phases. However, the increase in urinary calcium levels was not compensated by a commensurate increase in intestinal calcium absorption. Urinary deoxypyridinoline and N-telopeptide (markers of bone resorption and turnover that are often measured when testing for osteoporosis) trended upward, but the changes did not reach statistical significance. However, serum osteocalcin (a protein found in bone and important for the growth of bones and teeth) decreased significantly. The Atkins diet also significantly decreased urinary citrate, an inhibitor of calcium stone formation. The researchers concluded a very-low-carbohydrate diet *"delivers a marked acid load to the kidney, increases the risk for stone formation, decreases estimated calcium balance, and may increase the risk for bone loss."*[31]

This was a short study that did not measure long-term changes in bone mass or density. Nonetheless, the findings warrant caution and suggest that the findings of the aforementioned review by Kerstetter et al should not be extrapolated to high-protein diets with very low carbohydrate contents.

Conclusion

None of the common attacks on animal fats or protein hold up when subjected to close scientific scrutiny. These attacks are typically made out of sheer ignorance or in order to fulfil a hidden agenda (most commonly, promotion of vegan/vegetarian dietary dogmas). Either way, the basis for such attacks is not a sound one. Believe them at your own peril.

This bonus chapter has been excerpted from Anthony's acclaimed book The Fat Loss Bible, *available through Amazon and Lulu.com*

References for Bonus Chapter "Are Protein and Animal Fats Dangerous?"

1. Colpo A. LDL Cholesterol: Bad" Cholesterol, or Bad Science? *Journal of American Physicians and Surgeons*, Fall, 2005; 10 (3): 83-89.
2. World Health Organization. *Cardiovascular diseases (CVDs), Fact sheet N°317*. Sep, 2011. Available online: http://www.who.int/mediacentre/factsheets/fs317/en/index.html
3. Gordon T, et al. Menopause and coronary disease: The Framingham Study. *Annals of Internal Medicine*, 1978; 89: 157-161.
4. Writing Group for the Women's Health Initiative. Risks and Benefits of Estrogen Plus Progestin in Healthy Postmenopausal Women: Principal Results From the Women's Health Initiative Randomized Controlled Trial. *Journal of the American Medical Association*, Jul 17, 2002; 288 (3): 321-333.
5. Grady D, et al. Cardiovascular Disease Outcomes During 6.8 Years of Hormone Therapy: Heart and Estrogen/Progestin Replacement Study Follow-up (HERS II). *Journal of the American Medical Association*, Jul 3, 2002; 288 (1): 49-57.
6. The Women's Health Initiative Steering Committee. Effects of conjugated equine estrogen in postmenopausal women with hysterectomy: the Women's Health Initiative randomized controlled trial. *Journal of the American Medical Association*, 2004; 291: 1701-1712.

7. Petursson H, et al. Is the use of cholesterol in mortality risk algorithms in clinical guidelines valid? Ten years prospective data from the Norwegian HUNT 2 study. *Journal of Evaluation in Clinical Practice*, Sep 25, 2011. doi: 10.1111/j.1365-2753.2011.01767.x.
8. Cook JD, et al. Evaluation of the iron status in a population. *Blood*, 1976; 48: 449-455.
9. Jehn M, et al. Serum ferritin and risk of the metabolic syndrome in U.S. Adults. *Diabetes Care*, 2004; 27: 2422-2428.
10. Zacharski LR, et al. The iron (Fe) and atherosclerosis study (FeAST): a pilot study of reduction of body iron stores in atherosclerotic peripheral vascular disease. *American Heart Journal*, 2000; 139: 337-345.
11. Zacharski LR, et al. Reduction of Iron Stores and Cardiovascular Outcomes in Patients With Peripheral Arterial Disease: A Randomized Controlled Trial. *Journal of the American Medical Association*, 2007; 297: 603-610.
12. Zacharski LR, et al. Decreased cancer risk after iron reduction in patients with peripheral arterial disease: results from a randomized trial. *Journal of the National Cancer Institute*, Jul 16, 2008; 100 (14): 996-1002.
13. Fraser GE. Associations between diet and cancer, ischemic heart disease, and all-cause mortality in non-Hispanic white California Seventh-day Adventists. *American Journal of Clinical Nutrition*, Sept. 1999; 70 (3): 532S-538S.
14. Phillips RL. Role of lifestyle and dietary habits in risk of cancer among Seventh-Day Adventists. *Cancer Research*, Nov. 1975; 35: 3513-3522.
15. Thorogood M, et al. Risk of death from cancer and ischaemic heart disease in meat and non-meat eaters. *British Medical Journal*, Jun, 1994; 308: 1667-1670.
16. Key TJ, et al. Dietary habits and mortality in 11 000 vegetarians and health conscious people: results of a 17 year follow up. *British Medical Journal*, Sept 28, 1996; 313 (7060): 775-779.

17. Key TJ, et al. Mortality in British vegetarians: results from the European Prospective Investigation into Cancer and Nutrition (EPIC-Oxford). *American Journal of Clinical Nutrition*, 2009; 89 (Suppl): 1613S–1619S.

18. Key TJ, et al. Mortality in British vegetarians: review and preliminary results from EPIC-Oxford. *American Journal of Clinical Nutrition*, 2003; 78: 533S-538S.

19. Key TJ, et al. Cancer incidence in vegetarians: results from the European Prospective Investigation into Cancer and Nutrition (EPIC-Oxford). *American Journal of Clinical Nutrition*, 2009 89: (Suppl): 1620S-1626S.

20. Chang-Claude J, et al. Mortality pattern of German vegetarians after 11 years of follow-up. *Epidemiology*, Sep, 1992; 3 (5): 395-401.

21. Chang-Claude J, et al. Dietary and lifestyle determinants of mortality among German vegetarians. *International Journal of Epidemiology*, Apr, 1993; 22 (2): 228-236.

22. Enstrom JE. Health practices and cancer mortality among active California Mormons. *Journal of the National Cancer Institute*, Dec 6, 1989; 81 (23): 1807-1814.

23. Enstrom JE, et al. The relationship between vitamin C intake, general health practices, and mortality in Alameda County, California. *American Journal of Public Health*, Sep, 1986; 76 (9): 1124-1130.

24. Poortmans JR, Dellalieux O. Do regular high protein diets have potential health risks on kidney function in athletes? *International Journal of Sports Nutrition and Exercise Metabolism*, Mar. 2000; 10 (1): 28-38.

25. Blum M, et al. Protein intake and kidney function in humans: Its effect on normal aging. *Archives of Internal Medicine*, 1989; 149 (1): 211-212.

26. Facchini FS, Saylor KL. A low-iron-available, polyphenol-enriched, carbohydrate-restricted diet to slow progression of diabetic nephropathy. *Diabetes*, May 2003; 52 (5): 1204-1209.

27. Kerstetter JE, et al. Dietary protein and skeletal health: a review of recent human research. *Current Opinion in Lipidology*, 2011; 22: 16–20.

28. Ho-Pham LT, et al. Effect of vegetarian diets on bone mineral density: a Bayesian meta-analysis. *American Journal of Clinical Nutrition*, 2009; 90: 943–950.

29. Smith AM. Veganism and osteoporosis: A review of the current literature. *International Journal of Nursing Practice*, 2006; 12: 302–306.

30. Mazess RB, Warren Mather W. Bone mineral content of North Alaskan Eskimos. *American Journal of Clinical Nutrition*, 1974; 27: 916-925.

31. Reddy ST, et al. Effect of low-carbohydrate high-protein diets on acid-base balance, stone-forming propensity, and calcium metabolism. *American Journal of Kidney Diseases*, Aug, 2002; 40 (2): 265-274.

About the Author

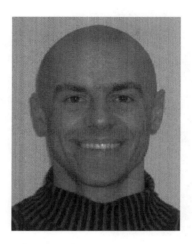

Anthony Colpo is a certified Physical Conditioning specialist, independent researcher and author hailing from Australia. Recently hailed as a "walking B.S. detector", he is well-known for his ability to systematically destroy even the most ingrained diet, training and health myths.

Having experienced first-hand the damaging effects of fad diets, Anthony is a strong critic of extreme eating approaches and advocates a non-dogmatic approach to nutrition. Rather than promote rigid, one-size-fits-all diets, Anthony believes nutritional plans should be tailored to an individual's needs, tastes, budget and lifestyle. He believes common-sense and sound science should always prevail above marketing and hyperbole.

He also maintains a keen interest in strength and conditioning research, which he uses to develop time-efficient programs for improving strength, muscle growth and cardiovascular fitness.

Anthony is the author of *The Fat Loss Bible* and *The Great Cholesterol Con*. An extensive collection of his highly informative, thought-provoking and often hilarious articles can be found at AnthonyColpo.com.

Made in the USA
Lexington, KY
28 April 2014